A HISTORY OF
MEDICINE *in*
50 OBJECTS

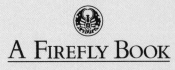

A FIREFLY BOOK

Published by Firefly Books Ltd. 2016

Copyright © 2016 Quid Publishing

First printing

Publisher Cataloging-in-Publication Data (U.S.)

Names: Paul, Gill, author.
Title: A history of medicine in 50 objects / Gill Paul.
Description: Richmond Hill, Ontario, Canada : Firefly Books, 2016.
| Includes bibliography and index. | Summary: "… A fascinating account of the physicians and scientists through the ages who identified specific problems affecting human health and set their minds to solving them. The objects are listed chronologically from prehistory to the present century, and include a Neolithic trepanned skull…; clay tablets from the Library of…; the red ribbon for AIDS awareness…; and thought-controlled prosthetic limbs… The book is illustrated in color and black and white with archive photographs and reproductions of art, maps, and line drawings" — Provided by publisher.
Identifiers: ISBN 978-1-77085-718-6 (hardcover)
Subjects: LCSH: Medicine – History.
Classification: LCC R131.P385 | DDC 610.9 – dc23

Library and Archives Canada Cataloguing in Publication

Paul, Gill, 1960-, author
    A history of medicine in 50 objects / Gill Paul.
Includes bibliographical references and index.
ISBN 978-1-77085-718-6 (bound)
    1. Medicine—History—Popular works. 2. Medical instruments and apparatus. 3. Medical supplies. 4. Material culture. I. Title. II. Title: History of medicine in fifty objects.
R133.P38 2016   610.9   C2016-900571-2

Published in the United States by
Firefly Books (U.S.) Inc.
P.O. Box 1338, Ellicott Station
Buffalo, New York 14205

Published in Canada by
Firefly Books Ltd.
50 Staples Avenue, Unit 1
Richmond Hill, Ontario L4B 0A7

Cover design: Erin R. Holmes

Interior design: Lindsey Johns

Printed in China

DEDICATION

For my dad, Professor John P. Paul, a bioengineer whose work greatly improved hip and knee joint replacements

Cover images
Front (left to right):
Wellcome Library, London, plantillustrations.org, Archives of Bayer AG *(top)*, Shutterstock.com/ Richard M Lee (btm) / Suzan Oschmann;
Back (left): Shutterstock.com/ nav; (right) /Olha Rohulya

Conceived, designed and produced by Quid Publishing
Level 4, Sheridan House
114 Western Road
Hove BN3 1DD
England

A HISTORY OF
MEDICINE *in*
50 OBJECTS

Gill Paul

FIREFLY BOOKS

Contents

Harvey's Diagram of Blood Circulation, page 72

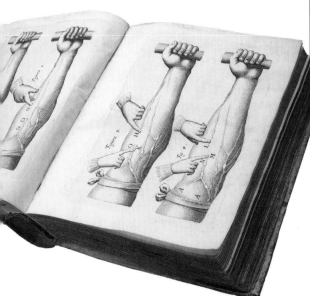

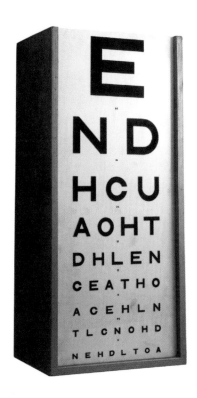

The Snellen Eye Chart, page 120

Introduction

The history of medicine is a riveting story of physicians and scientists through the ages who identified specific problems affecting human health and set their minds to solving them. Most new discoveries came about by building on the work of predecessors (it has been called "standing on the shoulders of giants"), like William Harvey did when he described the circulation of blood. Others took a leap into the unknown, such as Antonie van Leeuwenhoek, who found tiny objects he called "animalcules" when he peered at a drop of water through his special magnifying lenses. Many such pioneers were disbelieved or mocked at first, but fortunately for us they had the tenacity to pursue their hunches and chip away at a problem for decades without becoming discouraged.

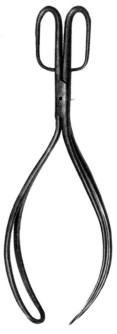

The invention of obstetric forceps by the Chamberlens in the 17th century helped to decrease the mortality rate in childbirth.

This book begins several millennia ago, when early humans believed disease was caused by evil spirits. It looks at the development of learning in Egypt and the Persian caliphates, in India, China, ancient Greece and Rome, and describes how the influence of Galen's teachings about the four "humors" held back progress in medicine for centuries. When plague swept the world between the 14th and the 17th centuries, physicians had no answers and the medical profession fell into disrepute, but the pendulum swung back once scientific methods were applied to research from the 17th century onward.

Some of the treatments endured by the sick were barbaric and must almost certainly have caused an agonizing death; the vast majority were simply ineffective. It wasn't until the 18th century that real progress was made in treating killer diseases, such as malaria and smallpox. Key developments in the 19th century were the

Hippocrates, the ancient Greek physician who set out doctors' obligations to their patients in his famous oath (see facing page).

> *Wherever the art of medicine is loved,*
> *there is also a love of humanity.*
> **—HIPPOCRATES, FIFTH CENTURY BCE**

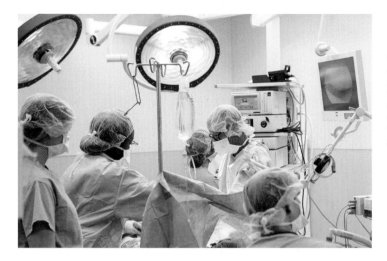

The modern operating environment bears little resemblance to the nonsterile, tiered theater or amphitheater in which students and other spectators once gathered to observe surgeons perform operations.

invention of anesthesia and antiseptics that made surgery safer, and the gradual discrediting of the "miasma" theory (which held that "bad air" caused disease) in favor of the more enlightened germ theory.

Throughout the 20th century, one by one diseases that had previously been death sentences became curable, either thanks to the "wonder drug" penicillin or through the World Health Organization's vaccination programs. By the end of the 20th century and the beginning of the 21st, medicine was changing every year, with exciting developments, in particular, in microsurgery, stem cell research, and nanotechnology—but still some diseases, such as HIV/AIDS, remain stubbornly incurable and rising antibiotic resistance threatens the spread of new killer bugs.

In choosing 50 key objects to illustrate the whole history of medicine thought there are inevitably some gaps, but the broad sweep of thinking is represented and the backbone of the story told. It's an incredible tale of the ingenuity of thousands of pioneering men and women who devoted their lives to making the world a healthier place.

I swear by Apollo the physician and Aesculapius and Health and All-heal and all the gods and goddesses, that, according to my ability and judgment, I will keep this Oath and this stipulation: to reckon him who taught me this Art equally dear to me as my parents, to share my substance with him and relieve his necessities, if required; to look upon his offspring on the same footing as my own brothers, and to teach them this art, if they shall wish to learn it, without fee or stipulation; and that by precept, lecture and every other mode of instruction, I will impart a knowledge of the Art to my own sons and those of my teachers and to disciples bound by a stipulation and oath according to the law of medicine, but to none others.

—THE HIPPOCRATIC OATH, CA. 400 BCE

Neolithic Trepanned Skulls

LOCATION:	Worldwide
DATE:	10,000–2,000 BCE
FIELD:	Surgery, psychiatry

Between 5 and 10 percent of Neolithic (late Stone Age) skulls found by archaeologists have one or more holes drilled in them, a procedure that later came to be known as trepanation or trephination. Trepanned skulls have been discovered all over South America, North Africa, Asia, Europe, New Zealand and the South Sea Islands, and it is the oldest surgical procedure for which evidence has been found. The reasons why it was carried out seem to vary. Some of the skulls show signs of head wounds, so the operation was probably performed to remove fractured pieces of bone. In other cases, it may have been used to release evil spirits that were thought to be causing headaches or insanity, and it may also have been a way of trying to bring the dead back to life.

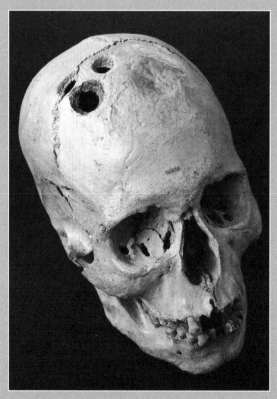

Truly it does not appear to me what certainty we may expect from the Scull being opened where it pains.

—THOMAS WILLIS, *THE LONDON PRACTICE OF PHYSICK*, 1685

THE NEOLITHIC WORLD VIEW

The earliest human beings were nomadic hunter-gatherers who moved from place to place in search of food. Men lived to an average of 35 years of age, whereas women lived to 30, and they were both relatively tall, with good teeth. By 8000 BCE they were beginning to settle into communities and develop an agricultural way of life, growing crops and keeping cows and sheep, and we can tell their diet was not so varied and protein-rich as in the nomadic years, because their height decreased. They also came into contact with more diseases, picking them up from itinerant traders and passing them on to each other in the insanitary living conditions in their settlements.

We can tell from their cave paintings and clay pottery that Neolithic humans believed in gods and omens, evil spirits and good-luck charms. They thought pain and disease were caused by evil spirits, and their shamans accordingly performed exorcism ceremonies on sick people. Trepanation may have been used to treat all kinds of disorders of the head, from epilepsy and migraines to mental-health issues, such as depression and schizophrenia.

The pieces of bone removed from the skull could measure as much as 1 to 2 inches (2.5–5 cm) in diameter, and they seem to have been kept as talismans against evil spirits; they may have been worn as a necklace. Large numbers of trepanned skulls found near military forts indicate that warriors may have extracted pieces of skull bone from their enemies for this purpose. According to anecdotal evidence quoted in ancient texts, some shamans advocated pulverizing the bone and mixing it with drinks, which were then consumed for extra protection against evil.

Early trepanations were most often carried out on adult males, but women and children could also be operated on. Patients remained conscious during the procedure.

Early Trepanation Techniques

The earliest trepanned skulls date from long before the introduction of metallurgy, and the holes were cut with sharp-edge flint knives or scraped with flint scrapers. Bow drills, in which a drill bit was tied to a wooden bow by means of a leather thong, came into use between 5000 and 4000 BCE. These produced a circular hole in the skull, whereas knives made rectangular or square ones. Copper and bronze were developed around 4250 BCE, and Aztec trepanation tools were made of bronze and gold. Some ancient Peruvian ones were made of obsidian (volcanic glass). Frequently the hole was left open, but in other cases it was covered with a piece of gourd, shell or even a plate of gold or silver.

THE FASHION FOR TREPANATION

The dangers of trepanation in the days before anesthesia and antisepsis are obvious: it could cause severe bleeding at the wound site, the patient could go into shock and there was a risk of brain swelling, blood clots and a danger of infection of the wound. However, it seems the early practitioners understood that they must not puncture the brain matter, and that explains the reasonably good survival rates. Around two-thirds of the holes found in Neolithic skulls show signs of healing, which indicates that the patients survived the procedure.

The operation was fashionable in ancient Egypt, the Roman Empire, among Celtic tribes and in ancient China, as well as among the Maya, Inca and Aztec civilizations of Central and South America and some North African peoples. Hippocrates (see pages 26–29) gave detailed instructions on performing trepanation in the case of head wounds. As well as allowing the removal of bone splinters, it would permit the draining of stagnant blood, which, he believed, would decay into pus if left.

Greek clinician Aretaeus of Cappadocia wrote around 150 CE about the use of trepanning as a treatment for epilepsy. In the Middle Ages it was seen as a way of releasing "bad air" or "evil vapors" from the skull and was also recommended for mania or melancholy. Dutch painter Hieronymus Bosch painted a trepanation being performed on a "simpleton" in his picture *The Cure for Madness* (late 15th century CE), although art historians differ on whether he is recommending the procedure or commenting on the folly of it. Some subjects had multiple operations: it is reported that Prince Philip of Orange (1554–1618) was trepanned 17 times by his surgeon.

Surgical instruments for trepanation included drills with cylindrical bits, a circular trephine (shown here in use) for cutting out a round piece of skull and forceps to remove extraneous matter.

> *If all means fail the last remedy is to open the fore part of the Skul with a Trepan, at a distance from sutures, that the evil air may breath out. By this means many desperate Epilepsies have been cured, and it may be safely done if the Chyrurgoen be skilful.*
> —LAZARUS RIVERIUS, *THE PRACTICE OF PHYSICK*, 1655

As a cure for epilepsy or madness, trepanning can have done no good; but those, such as the Kissii of Kenya, who used it as a treatment for headaches after a head injury, were onto something. It may well have been an effective treatment if it relieved intracranial pressure due to a brain hemorrhage or swelling.

MODERN USES OF TREPANATION TECHNIQUES

Some types of brain surgery are still performed through holes in the skull; the operation is now known as a craniotomy. Modern cutting tools, coated in diamond, have come a long way from the flint knives of Neolithic times, and the piece of bone removed is almost always replaced. One of the most common modern uses of craniotomy is to monitor intracranial pressure after a head injury or a stroke, but it can also be carried out to allow surgeons to remove brain tumors, to take clear neurological images and to insert stimulators that can help people with Parkinson's disease and epilepsy. In other words, some of the trepanners of previous millennia were working along the right lines.

Voluntary Trepanation

Bart Huges was a Dutch librarian who had studied medicine in Amsterdam without graduating. He argued in evolutionary terms that once man began to walk upright his brain circulation dropped, and that trepanation could help the brain to function more effectively by creating an optimum balance between blood and spinal fluid. He published his theory in 1964 and, practicing what he preached, in 1965 he performed a trepanation on himself using a foot-operated dentist's drill. The operation took just 45 minutes. When he went to a local hospital for an x-ray to prove what he had done, they admitted him to a psychiatric ward, but that did not stop dozens of others from following in his footsteps. There are now many Internet sites that advocate trepanation and even give instructions on how to perform it. Needless to say, it is not recommended.

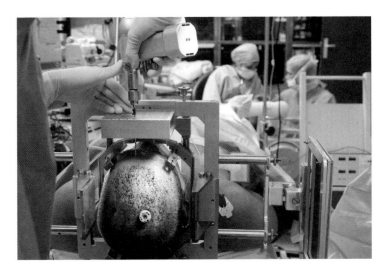

A modern surgeon drills a hole in the skull of a patient who has Parkinson's disease to stimulate an area deep inside the brain. The procedure helps to reduce tremor.

The Edwin Smith Papyrus

LOCATION:	Egypt
DATE:	3000 BCE
FIELD:	Neurosurgery, orthopedics

In 1862 American archaeologist Edwin Smith bought a scroll from a couple of dealers in a market in Luxor, Egypt. It was 15 feet (4.5 m) long and written in the hieratic script used by ancient Egyptian priests, which Smith was not able to decipher. When a translation was finally produced in the 1920s, it was found to be a compelling document describing medical and surgical procedures for treating 48 different ailments. Experts judged it to be the work of a scribe living about 1600 BCE, copying an original papyrus that dated from about 2500–3000 BCE. This made it the oldest known surgical text. But astonishingly, some of the knowledge it contained was more advanced than that of Hippocrates, who lived in Greece more than two millennia later—and a few of the procedures it described are still performed in the present day.

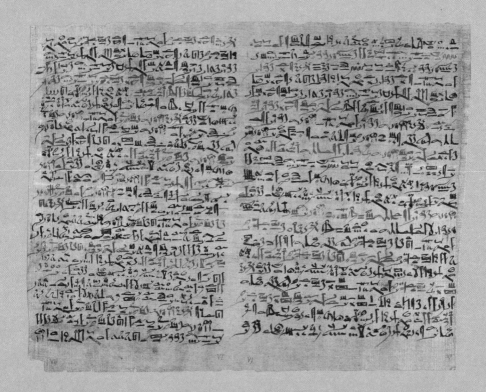

THE FIRST PHYSICIAN

The people who settled in the Nile Valley believed in evil spirits that caused floods, pestilence and misfortune, and they had a complex range of rituals and incantations for their gods that were designed to ward off such evil. From about 3000 BCE they developed hieroglyphics and recorded long scripts on a range of topics. The first pyramid was built as a dead pharaoh's tomb about 2700 BCE, and mummification was practiced from the same period to make sure of safe passage to the next world.

During the 27th century BCE, there lived a remarkable man by the name of Imhotep. He was chancellor to Pharaoh Djoser, and he was also a royal architect and engineer who may have been responsible for designing the first step pyramid at Saqqara. He was a high priest and a renowned physician, and some speculate that he was the author of the Edwin Smith Papyrus, with its rational approach to diagnosis and treatment. Imhotep's many talents were greatly respected by his contemporaries and he became the only nonroyal to be granted divine status after death. He is certainly the first physician whose name lives on to the present day. However, critics of the theory that he authored the papyrus point out that it deals mainly with battlefield injuries and Imhotep was not a battlefield surgeon.

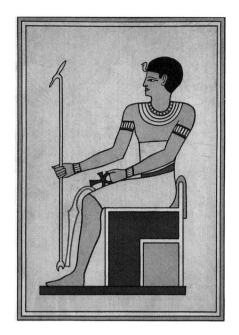

Imhotep was born a commoner but worked his way up to become Pharaoh Djoser's second-in-command. He is the first physician thought to have rejected magic spells in favor of herbal potions for treating disease.

THE 48 AILMENTS

Of the 48 ailments listed in the Edwin Smith Papyrus, 27 concern head injuries and six deal with trauma to the spine. Each entry follows the same structure. First the injury is described and then tips are given on the examination of the patient. This includes questions to be asked of the patient, pulses taken and observations on skin and eye color, nasal secretions and stiffness of joints. Next comes the diagnosis, and one of three prognoses is given for each: it will be listed as "An ailment I can treat," "An ailment I shall contend with" or "An ailment not to be treated"—in other words, one for which the author knew of no cure. Thereafter it describes the treatment to be given. There are some glosses or notes at the end, that seem to have been added a few hundred years after the original text.

> *In medical knowledge Egypt leaves the rest of the world behind.*
> **—HOMER, THE ODYSSEY, CA. 800 BCE**

Among the remarkable aspects of the papyrus are the detailed descriptions of the brain, and it shows the author's understanding of the brain and spinal cord and how damage to different areas could cause paralysis, incontinence, aphasia and seizures. It is surprising, because Egyptians believed the seat of the emotions and thought was in the heart and thought so little of the brain that it was discarded during mummification. Four thousand years before William Harvey described circulation (see pages 72–75), the author of the papyrus knew that blood moved in vessels with the heart at their center. In Case 25, he describes the same procedure for treating a dislocated jaw that is followed today. In Case 48, he describes a test for irritation of the lumbar or sciatic

Mummification

Ancient Egyptians considered it vital that the dead were preserved so that the body would be ready for resurrection in the next life. The first step in mummification was to force the brain out through the nostrils with an iron hook, before the heart and other internal organs were removed and dried. The organs were elaborately wrapped and stored in "canopic" jars near where the body would lie, then the heart was placed back inside the cadaver before it was embalmed and wrapped in bandages. This procedure gave Egyptians some knowledge of anatomical dissection, and the mummies they left behind offer modern paleopathologists an insight into the illnesses they experienced. Rheumatoid arthritis was common, as were bladder and kidney stones, gout, gallstones and atherosclerosis (fatty deposits in the arteries; see page 191). There is no sign of rickets and little dental decay, indicating a decent diet, and so far no mummy has been found to have syphilis.

Bronze and copper mummification knives, 600–200 BCE, used to remove internal organs.

Corpses were wrapped in fine linen, with amulets between the layers, and a scroll of the Book of the Dead *was placed between the hands.*

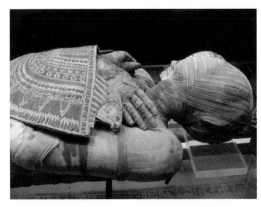

nerve by getting the patient to raise and lower their straight legs; this is today known as Lasègue's test, after a French physician of the 19th century.

Many of the treatments described would have had a good chance of success. Wounds were to be bound in fresh meat, which had hemostatic properties (that is, it helped to control bleeding). Honey, which has antibiotic properties, might be applied and opiates were given for pain relief. Case 30, shown here, describes the use of meat and honey for a neck sprain. A cream used for removing wrinkles contained urea, which is an ingredient of many modern anti-wrinkle creams.

SCIENCE, NOT MAGIC

Apart from one entry on the reverse side of the scroll giving advice on transforming an old man into a youth, the Edwin Smith Papyrus is remarkably devoid of magic. Trepanation is not mentioned once, and there is no advice on exorcising evil spirits. The author occasionally uses similes to clarify his description—for example, he compares the fork at the head of the ramus in the mandible (the lower jawbone) to the claw of a two-toed bird—but he does not include spells.

In comparison, the Ebers Papyrus of ca. 1550 BCE has more than 700 magical and folk remedies to cure ailments that range from crocodile bites and toenail pain to infestations of flies, rats and scorpions. It lists 21 ways to deal with coughs, 29 types of eye diseases, 18 skin complaints and 15 diseases of the abdomen; and the "cures" include the application of herbal remedies plus incantations to the relevant god or goddess.

The anonymous author of the Edwin Smith Papyrus has all the hallmarks of a modern scientist, searching for evidence he can see with his own eyes and using logic to reach his conclusions.

Case 30

Title: **Instructions concerning a sprain in a vertebra of his neck.**

Examination: **If thou examinest a man having a sprain in a vertebra of his neck, thou shouldst say to him: "Look at thy two shoulders and thy breast." When he does so, the seeing possible to him is painful.**

Diagnosis: **Thou shouldst say concerning him: "One having a sprain in a vertebra of his neck. An ailment which I will treat."**

Treatment: **Thou shouldst bind it with fresh meat the first day. Now afterward thou shouldst treat [with] ywrw [unidentified] [and] honey every day until he recovers.**

Gloss: **As for: "a sprain" he is speaking of a rending of two members [although each] is [still] in its place.**

This recognition of the localization of function in the brain ... shows an astonishing early discernment which has been more developed by modern surgeons only within the present generations.
—JAMES HENRY BREASTED, TRANSLATOR OF THE EDWIN SMITH PAPYRUS, 1930

Clay Tablets from Mesopotamia

LOCATION:	Mesopotamia (roughly modern-day Iraq and Syria)
DATE:	Seventh century BCE
FIELD:	Pharmacology, surgery

King Ashurbanipal reigned from 668 to 627 BCE, and during that time, he built in the city of Nineveh a royal library containing up to 30,000 clay tablets, making it one of the largest of his day. The subjects covered included divination, astronomy and literature (the *Epic of Gilgamesh* was one of the texts), and there were also about 660 stones describing medical knowledge through the previous centuries. These tablets were excavated only in the mid-19th century and it took some time to translate their cuneiform texts, but when they were made available, scholars were stunned to discover how modern and comparatively rational the medical thinking was.

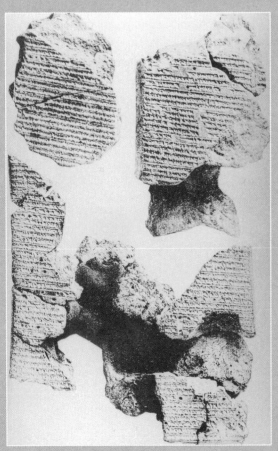

If a physician has performed a major operation on a lord with a bronze lancet and has saved the lord's life ... he shall receive 10 shekels of silver .... If a physician performed a major operation on a lord ... and has caused the lord's death ... they shall cut off his hand.

—HAMMURABI CODE, CA. 1695 BCE

SORCERERS AND SURGEONS

From the tablets of Ashurbanipal we learn that the sick were treated by sorcerers known as *ashipu*, who diagnosed ailments and used charms and incantations to drive demons from the afflicted, as well as physicians known as *asu*, who used a combination of herbal medicines and surgery. Long lists of diagnoses are organized from head to toe in the tablets, with separate sections for convulsive disorders, gynecology and pediatrics. They tell us, for example, that the Mesopotamians knew that diseases, such as syphilis, were sexually transmitted, and they understood how to extract essential oils from plants.

Unlike the Egyptians, they believed in bathing wounds, either in hot water or beer, and they made poultices from a variety of ingredients, including prunes, lizard dung and the dregs from a bottle of wine. Some recipes for plasters involved heating plant resin or animal fat with an alkaline substance, which would have formed a kind of soap with antibacterial properties.

Among the herbal remedies we can identify, many had antibiotic and antiseptic properties and some, such as their remedy for excessive bleeding, are essentially the same as the modern remedies for the same condition.

The Hammurabi Code of ca. 1695 BCE set out laws governing all kinds of contractual matters, from family affairs through to tradesmen's pay and conditions—including those of surgeons. The punishments for poor performance were linked to the status of the client.

The Hammurabi Code

A Babylonian tablet, written about 1695 BCE, that, among other tenets, laid down the conditions under which physicians worked and stated that they would receive decent pay for their services. There do not appear to have been any penalties for prescribing the wrong medicine or failing to cure a patient, but if the patient died during surgery, there were sanctions according to his or her rank. If an important person died, the surgeon's hand would be cut off, but if a slave died under the knife, the surgeon need only supply a new slave.

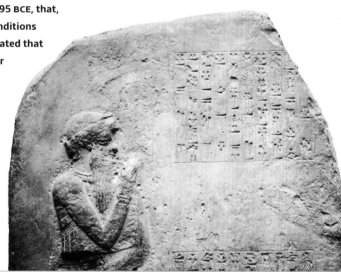

Atharva Veda

LOCATION: India

DATE: Sixth century BCE – seventh century CE

FIELD: Medicine, surgery, obstetrics, pediatrics, psychiatry, surgery, toxicology, geriatrics, ophthalmology, plastic surgery

According to Hindu legend, Lord Dhanvantari, the founder of the Ayurvedic system of medicine, is an incarnation of Lord Vishnu and he received his medical knowledge direct from Brahma, the god of Creation. Dhanvantari created many herbal cures and natural remedies, which are listed in the *Atharva Veda*, and was also said to be a skilled surgeon. The sick still pray for cures at temples dedicated to him across India, but the influence of Ayurveda has extended far beyond Indian shores. Some call it the world's most ancient medical science and claim that it influenced Tibetan, Chinese and Greek medicine, making it "the mother of all healing."

> It is not possible to see with the physical eyes the subtle principle of the spirit in the body, for it is visible to the eye of wisdom or meditation alone. The wise physician therefore should know the truth by studying the body as well as the text of the science
>
> —SUSHRUTA, CA. FIRST CENTURY BCE

THE SOURCE OF AYURVEDIC LEARNING

The wisdom of Brahma was passed down through the centuries in four ancient Sanskrit texts, known as Vedas. One of these, the *Atharva Veda*, thought to have been transcribed by several authors between the sixth century BCE and the seventh century CE, consists of 114 hymns and incantations to cure disease. Two supplementary texts, the *Charaka Samhita* and the *Sushruta Samhita*, were added later. Together, they formed a systematic classification of diseases, their symptoms and descriptions of their cures. By 400 CE the texts had been translated into Chinese and there were signs of their influence appearing in Chinese medical practice (see pages 22–25). It has also been suggested that their theory of three *doshas* was picked up by travelers and taken back to ancient Greece, where it was the origin of the theory of the four humors (see pages 26–29).

Modern Ayurvedic practitioners still follow a system that was established in the Vedas. They believe in a balance in the body, and place emphasis on spirituality and emotional stability as well as physical well-being. To have good health, harmony between thoughts, feelings and physical actions must be in balance. Illness can be caused when, for example, patients misjudge situations, or use the sense organs inappropriately, bringing about an imbalance in their three doshas, or energies: *vatha*, *pitha* and *kapha*.

THE DOSHAS

According to Ayurvedic belief, the five elements—ether, air, fire, water and earth—are forever changing and interacting in our universe. When in balance, they sustain life, but when out of balance they cause illness. These elements are the building blocks of the three doshas, and each human being has a unique ratio of them, like a DNA fingerprint, which is determined at conception.

Cures at the Dhanvantari Temple

Devotees of Ayurveda still meditate and pray at the second-century BCE Dhanvantari temple in Kerala to cure problems caused by imbalances in the doshas. Specific parts of the temple complex have their own purposes. Those with eye diseases seek help at the Nelluvai temple. The Guruvayur temple offers relief from rheumatic diseases; an offering or *Mukkudi* made of Ayurvedic herbs, when offered to the deities and then imbibed by devotees, is said to cure all kinds of abdominal and gastric disorders, and bathing in the pond on the north side of the temple gives mental purity and a healthy body. Physicians perform devotions at the temple to make sure of favorable outcomes for their patients, and there is now an Ayurvedic hospital and research center on the site.

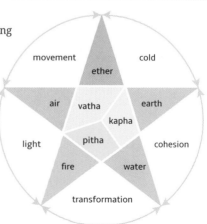

- Vatha energy is dynamic and mobile, and it governs respiration, circulation, elimination, movement, speech, the nervous system, creativity and enthusiasm. An excess of vatha can cause constipation, arthritis and anxiety.

- Pitha energy is transformative and intelligent, and it governs digestion, the metabolism, temperature, the complexion, courage, cheerfulness, and intellect. Excess pitha can cause inflammation, infections and ulcers.

> *When diet is wrong, medicine is of no use; when diet is correct, medicine is of no need.*
> —AYURVEDIC PROVERB

- Kapha energy is structural and physical, and it governs growth, the balance and excretion of bodily fluids, potency, patience, compassion and understanding. Excess kapha can cause weight gain, diabetes and congestive disorders.

Typically, one or two doshas will dominate in a person, so an individual might be vatha, vatha/pitha, pitha/kapha and so forth. There are seven main "dosha types," with different dosha combinations, and each of these has specific areas that tend to go out of balance and cause disease. An Ayurvedic practitioner seeks to determine the patient's dosha type to strengthen the natural balance of their basic constitution, because that is the best defense against illness.

AYURVEDIC DIAGNOSIS

An Ayurvedic practitioner will ask each patient detailed questions about their diet, lifestyle, likes and dislikes, bowel movements and urinary function, general health and parents' health to work out the dominant dosha or doshas and build up a picture of where imbalances might lie. They will assess the patient's appearance (shape, size and posture), speech and movement, and they will examine the eyes, tongue and even the lines on the face. Taking the pulse is an all-important diagnostic tool, and this is done at three points on each wrist. The diagnoses do not resemble those in Western medicine, because practitioners look for toxic imbalances in the doshas, and they believe diseases develop in six distinct stages, each leading to the next if not healed in the meantime.

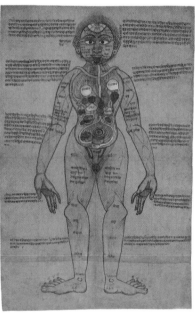

A drawing, ca. 1800, that sets out human anatomy as understood by Ayurvedic physicians. Instead of focusing on physical characteristics, the emphasis is on the function of the different organs and systems and the way they interact.

Some remedies suggested in early Ayurvedic literature conform with modern medical thinking in the West. For example, consuming raw goat liver is recommended to treat anemia following blood loss, and as recently as 1926, researchers George Minot and William Murphy confirmed that eating liver was indeed an effective way of treating anemia.

REMEDIES AND TREATMENTS

Ayurvedic treatments are administered differently for those of different dosha types and can take the form of *panchakarma* (elimination), *shamana* (pacification) and *bhrimana* (nourishing) therapies. Panchakarma might consist of a herbal oil massage or steam inhalation, and in previous centuries it could have consisted of laxatives, emetics and enemas to cleanse the digestive system. Panchakarma therapies are used for ailments involving gas, hormones, mucus and calcification, and by ridding the body of excesses, they leave room for it to rebalance itself. Bhrimana therapies address spirituality and might include yoga, meditation and mantras.

Localized complaints, such as a sprained ankle, would be treated with pacification therapies: diet and lifestyle modifications plus herbal remedies. A *sattvic* (pure) diet of seasonal fruits and vegetables with nonanimal proteins, which will not overburden the system, is generally recommended.

Ayurvedic practitioners in the ancient world excelled at surgery, and they had 121 different instruments designed for surgical purposes, such as draining fluid, treating cataracts, removing bladder and kidney stones and cauterizing wounds. Dissection was forbidden, but trainee surgeons practiced their skills on leather bags filled with slime or on pieces of meat.

Early Nose Jobs

Amputation of the nose was a common punishment in parts of ancient India. Ayurvedic doctors devised a method of reconstructing the nose by using a leaf-shape flap of skin from the forehead, which remained attached near the bridge of the nose. It was twisted around and pulled down over the nasal cavity, then sewn into place. Wooden tubes would be inserted so the patient could breathe while it was healing. When a report of this operation appeared in the London periodical *The Gentleman's Magazine* in 1794, European surgeons sailed to India to observe this early form of rhinoplasty and began to perform the operation back home (see pages 148–51).

Illustration accompanying an 1816 article on Indian rhinoplasty operations that were performed on two British army officers. The lost nose was replaced with tissue folded down from the officers' foreheads.

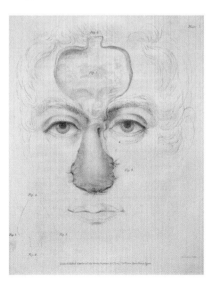

Huangchi Neijing

LOCATION: China
DATE: 475–300 BCE
FIELD: Traditional Chinese medicine

The earliest writings of the Chinese Shang dynasty (ca. 1600–1046 BCE) show a people who believed in divination and magic, and indicate that they thought illness was caused by curses placed on the living by their dead ancestors. It was a huge leap from there to the philosophy of balance and harmony in all things that is the foundation of the immensely influential *Huangchi Neijing*. Its authors identify the causes of illness as diet, lifestyle, the emotions, the environment and the patient's age, and they designed a chart showing the meridians in the body along which acupuncture needles could be inserted to relieve ailments. The lessons contained in this ancient text are still at the core of traditional Chinese medicine as it is practiced today.

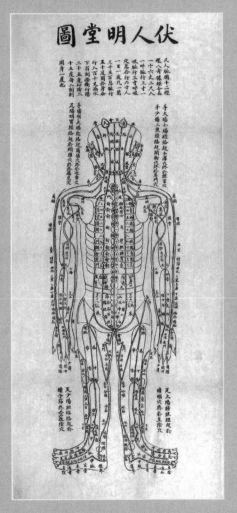

Health and well-being can be achieved only by remaining centered in spirit, guarding against the squandering of energy, promoting the constant flow of qi and blood, maintaining harmonious balance of yin and yang, adapting to the changing seasonal and yearly macrocosmic influences and nourishing one's self preventively. This is the way to a long and happy life.
—*HUANGCHI NEIJING*

THE GREAT HUANGDI

Emperor Huangdi (also known as the Yellow Emperor) is a legendary figure who is said to have reigned over the Chinese empire in the middle of the third millennium BCE. He was a child prodigy who became renowned for his great wisdom. Before his time, the Chinese lived nomadic lifestyles, but according to myth he introduced coins, government institutions, the bow sling, agriculture, carts, boats and musical instruments, among many other developments, making him the founder of civilization in China. Two thousand years after his reign, when scholars were writing a treatise on how to cure disease by creating balance in the body, they presented it as a question and answer session between the great Huangdi and six of his ministers. This may have been a strategy to avoid any repercussions for themselves in case the authorities disapproved of their work.

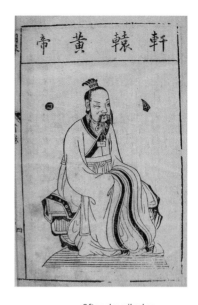

Often described as the first ruler of China, Emperor Huangdi (2698–2598 BCE) is said to have tamed wild animals, including bears, and made them fight in battle alongside his armies. Huangdi is also credited with many inventions that improved the lives of his people.

The *Huangchi Neijing* consists of two texts, each with 81 chapters: the first is known as *Suwen* (*Questions of an Organic and Fundamental Nature*) and sets out the theoretical basis of Chinese medicine and the techniques for diagnosis; the second text, *Lingshu* (*Spiritual Pivot*), explains the use of acupuncture in treating illness.

There have been many translations of *Huangchi Neijing* through the centuries, including one dating from the eighth century, with commentaries by Wang Bing, and another from the 11th century by Lin Yi. It is still read today and an influential new translation was published in 2011 by scholars at the Ludwig Maximilian University in Munich, Germany.

Taoism

The ancient philosopher and poet Laozi (or Lao-tzu; ca. sixth–fourth century BCE) is generally reckoned to have been the founder of the philosophy/religion of Taoism, and the author of the *Tao Te Ching*. The Tao (which means "way" or "path") is said to be the source of and the force behind everything that lives. By using a mixture of analogy and ancient sayings, the Tao Te Ching promotes a life lived according to the principles of virtue, humility and balance in all things. Followers of the Tao live in accordance with the rhythms of the seasons, the stars, and the sun and moon. The influence of Taoism was crucial in the development of Chinese medical practice.

DIAGNOSING IMBALANCES

The great achievement of the *Huangchi Neijing* was the development of the idea that health is influenced by a range of internal or external phenomena, which either stimulate or depress the life force. Disease can be caused by six excesses (listed in the text as wind, cold, fire/heat, dampness, dryness and summer heat) or seven emotions (joy, anger, anxiety, brooding, sorrow, fear and sudden fright). Each of these causes particular symptoms; summer heat, for example, causes sweating, dizziness and nausea.

Opposing forces—for example, light and dark—are complementary only if they exist in balance. This idea of balanced energies may have derived from Ayurvedic practice; but, rather than doshas, Chinese practitioners aim to restore balance between two forces in the body known as yin and yang, as well as between the five elements of earth, water, fire, wood and metal, which each relate to particular organs, to the senses, to colors, tastes and types of climate.

When diagnosing patients, the Chinese physician, like the Ayurvedic one, will check the patient's pulses, of which there are six in each wrist. There are various descriptions of pulses in the *Huangchi Neijing*, including "smooth as a flowing stream," "light as flicking the skin with a plume" or, ominously, "dead as a rock," and taking pulses is a skill that requires many years to master. Practitioners look at the color and size of a patient's tongue and check for signs of teeth marks or coating. They look at the eyes, smell the breath and body odor, listen to the breathing and the sound of the voice, and from these combined observations they can judge where weakness and imbalance lie.

Yin and Yang

Yin and yang are parts of a whole, and each requires the other. The qualities of yin are dark, moist, and female, whereas the qualities of yang are bright, dry, and male. In Chinese medicine, yin and yang must be in balance with each other and if one is deficient there is said to be a "vacuity." A vacuity of yin leads to symptoms such as dry mouth, dark urine, night sweats, insomnia, a red tongue with little fur, and a fine and rapid pulse. A vacuity of yang leads to cold limbs, a pale complexion, large quantities of clear urine, diarrhea, a pale, enlarged tongue, and a slightly weak, slow pulse.

A physician needs to possess a moral conscience, ethical conduct and a compassionate attitude toward those in need of attention. In all interactions with patients, the physician is always composed, takes the necessary time, remains objective and performs every procedure with the utmost care and precision.
—HUANGCHI NEIJING

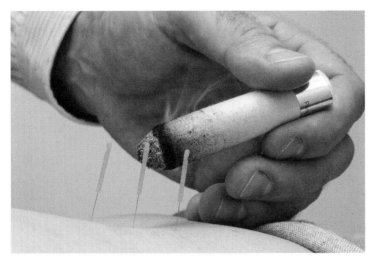

ACUPUNCTURE AND MOXIBUSTION

According to the *Huangchi Neijing*, there are 12 main meridians in the body, corresponding to the number of rivers in the ancient Chinese Empire, and along these flows a substance called chi, or qi, the life force. Each meridian corresponds to particular organs and bodily functions, and there are 365 acupuncture points located along them. By inserting fine needles at specific points, an acupuncturist stimulates the flow of qi and thus relieves the symptoms of illness.

Illustration from Routes of the Fourteen Meridians and their Functions, *written by the Chinese physician Hua Shou in the mid-14th century. It became a classic in the study of acupuncture.*

There are three chapters on pain in the *Huangchi Neijing*, including one on lower-back pain, and many of the meridians it describes seem to follow the pathways of referred pain we know about today. Referred pain is pain that is felt in a different part of the body from the actual disease or injury; for example, the pain from gallstones is often felt in the right shoulder blade. There was no knowledge of the nervous system in ancient China, because anatomical dissection was forbidden, so practitioners reached these conclusions purely by external observation.

Moxibustion is another treatment used in traditional Chinese medicine. A cone of moxa (the powdered roots of the mugwort plant, *Artemisia argyi*) is placed on the appropriate acupuncture point and set alight, and the heat created increases yang.

Acupuncture is widely practiced in the 21st century, and there is evidence that it can be effective for the treatment of headaches and chronic lower-back pain, although detractors claim it relies on the placebo effect (see page 139).

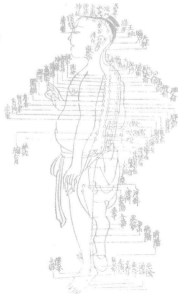

The Tree of Hippocrates

LOCATION: Greece
DATE: Fifth century BCE
FIELD: Medicine

[Hippocrates] is, above all, the exemplar of that flexible, critical, well-poised attitude of mind, always on the lookout for sources of error, which is the very essence of the scientific spirit.

—FIELDING GARRISON, *A SHORT HISTORY OF MEDICINE*, 1913

On the Greek island of Kos, a wise and learned teacher called Hippocrates (born ca. 460 BCE) used to instruct his students beneath the shade of a plane tree. Like the ancient Indians and Chinese, he believed that imbalance in the body caused illness, but he thought this imbalance lay in the four humors: blood, phlegm, yellow bile and black bile. More than 70 volumes of texts said to have been written by him were collected in the great library of Alexandria and called *The Hippocratic Corpus*. These would influence medical thought right up to the 19th century, and Hippocrates would be acclaimed as the "Father of Western Medicine."

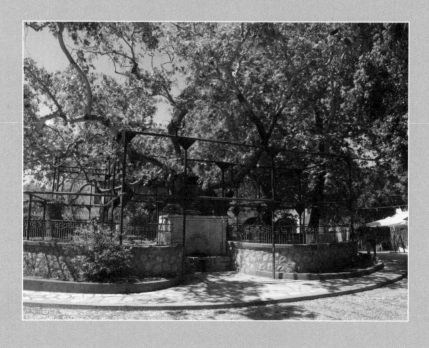

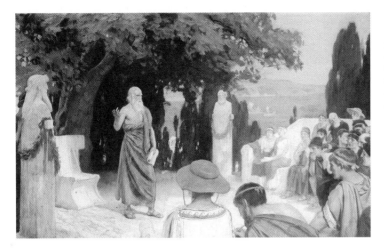

Hippocrates teaching his students under the original plane tree in Kos; he believed physicians should be strictly professional at all times, with a neat and well-groomed appearance and a calm and serious bedside manner.

THE MEDICAL SCHOOL ON KOS

Both Aristotle and Plato, writing in the fourth century BCE, mention Hippocrates and the first biography of him was written in the second century CE by Soranus of Ephesus. According to Soranus, Hippocrates' father and grandfather were both physicians and he trained at the Asklepeion on Kos, a temple dedicated to Asklepios, the god of physicians. Patients would sleep overnight in the temple and the following morning would describe their dreams to the priest, who would diagnose their ailments accordingly. One of the key medical developments attributed to Hippocrates was the separation of medicine and religion. He believed that illness was caused by external, physical factors, not by the gods, and sought to heal by promoting harmony within the body.

Hippocrates is said to have traveled far afield in his lifetime, teaching and practicing medicine, and he is credited with curing the king of Macedonia of tuberculosis. His age at death is variously given as 83, 85, 90 or well over 100. *The Hippocratic Corpus* is written in Ionic Greek and includes textbooks, lectures, essays and notes, all in random order. They are in different styles and at times contradict each other, leading modern scholars to conclude there were probably about 19 different authors.

The Library of Alexandria

The city of Alexandria in Egypt was founded in 331 BCE by Alexander the Great, and its great library was established by his successor, Ptolemy I Soter. It was tasked with collecting all the wisdom of the world, and at its height was said to contain as many as 700,000 volumes, which official scribes transcribed onto papyrus scrolls. Any ships that came into port had their books seized for the library, and when Athens lent the original works of some of its great writers, they were not returned. The library was part of a museum complex where scholars could study and give lectures on their discoveries, subsidized by public funds. It was burned down, although it is not clear whether the main destruction was from a fire started by Julius Caesar in 48 BCE, by Aurelian in the 270s CE or by Theophilus, Pope of Alexandria, in 391. Fortunately, *The Hippocratic Corpus* survived.

THE HIPPOCRATIC APPROACH TO HEALING

There were two schools of thought in ancient Greek medicine: the Knidian school, which saw the body as a collection of separate parts and focused on diagnosing the symptoms produced by dysfunction of one part; and the Koan school, which saw the body as a complete organism that should be treated holistically and aimed to provide patients with prognoses. *The Hippocratic Corpus* was very much of the latter school, arguing that disease was a natural process arising from disharmony and stating that the body has the power to rebalance the humors and heal itself, if given the right support by the physician.

Hippocrates' followers rarely used surgery; their methods were much more passive. Hippocrates himself is said to have prescribed the intake of a light diet (only liquids during fevers and the healing of wounds), gymnastics and other forms of exercise, massage, hydrotherapy and sea bathing. He believed in rest, keeping the patient in clean and sterile conditions, applying soothing balms (*enhemes*) composed of herbal and mineral mixtures, and the consumption of apple cider vinegar.

A Hippocratic bench was designed for the traction of broken limbs, and his techniques for treating dislocations of the hip and jaw were not surpassed until the 19th century. He was also ahead of his time in using tourniquets to stem bleeding and auscultation (listening to the heart and lungs) as an aid to diagnosis. The Hippocratic school used pipes to drain the chest wall in the case of abscesses and treated hemorrhoids with cauterization, excision, or ligation, but on the whole the style was noninterventionist.

HUMORAL THEORY

Humoral theory may have originated in ancient Egypt, but it was in Greece that it was first systematized. Proponents of the theory of the four humors believed that blood was produced by the liver, and that too much of it caused fevers; accordingly, bloodletting was used to rebalance the proportions of the humors. This technique was used even if the patient was hemorrhaging (although Hippocrates himself is said to have used it only rarely). An excess of yellow bile was said to produce aggression and anger, whereas black bile caused depression and phlegm caused apathy. Purging with laxatives or emetics might be

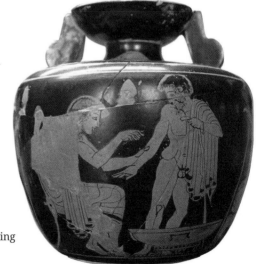

An ancient Greek flask depicting a patient's vein being opened to rebalance his humors. Humoral medicine was influential in the Western world for more than 2,000 years, until scientists were able to observe bacteria under microscopes in the mid-19th century.

prescribed (one of the emetics was the lethal poison hellebore), and suppuration of wounds was practiced to eliminate phlegm. Fasting was also recommended to prevent any increase in the humors.

Each humor was also associated with an element—air, fire, earth and water— and with a time of year; for example, yellow bile was associated with summer and caused warm diseases, whereas phlegm was associated with winter and caused cold diseases.

ON BEING A PHYSICIAN

Perhaps the most lasting legacy of the Hippocratic school was its lessons on being a good physician. Hippocrates taught that physicians should be well-kempt, serious, honest and direct with patients, always doing their best to help and above all causing no harm. They should observe closely the patient's pulse, complexion, excretions, pain and movements, and always take a full case history—a practice that died out after his day.

It is unlikely that the Hippocratic Oath was formulated by Hippocrates himself, but it would become his best-known legacy. It has been revised many times, but key parts of it are still used in medical oaths today, in particular, the clauses about preserving patient confidentiality, about respecting one's teachers and vowing to pass on medical research to others in the field, and treating the ill to the best of one's ability while avoiding doing any harm.

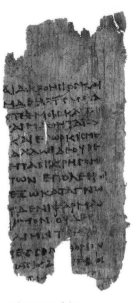

A fragment of the Hippocratic Oath, written on parchment in Ionic Greek. It may have been produced by one of Hippocrates' students, according to the principles he taught.

> *Whenever a doctor cannot do good, he must be kept from doing harm.*
> —HIPPOCRATES

Key Principles of the Original Hippocratic Oath

- I will apply dietetic measures for the benefit of the sick according to my ability and judgment; I will keep them from harm and injustice.
- I will neither give a deadly drug to any who asked for it, nor will I make a suggestion to this effect.
- I will give no woman a pessary to cause abortion.
- Whatever houses I may visit, I will come for the benefit of the sick, remaining free of all ... mischief and, in particular, of sexual relations with both male and female persons.
- What I may see or hear in the course of treatment ... in regard to the life of men ... I will keep to myself, holding such things to be shameful to be spoken about.
- If I fulfill this oath and do not violate it, may it be granted to me to enjoy life and art.

The Aqua Appia

LOCATION: Rome
DATE: 312 BCE
FIELD: Public health

The trial and proof of water are made as follows. If it be of an open and running stream, before we lay it on, the shape of the limbs of the inhabitants of the neighborhood should be looked to and considered. If they are strongly formed, of fresh color, with sound legs and without blear eyes, the supply is of good quality.

—SEXTUS JULIUS FRONTINUS, REPORT ON AQUEDUCT SYSTEM, END OF FIRST CENTURY CE

The Tiber River, which runs through Rome, used to contain everything from dead animals to the contents of citizens' chamber pots, and Romans were well aware that bathing in and drinking the water caused disease; but until the construction of the first aqueduct in 312 BCE, many had little choice. The Aqua Appia flowed for just over 10 miles (16 km), mostly underground, until it emerged in the city center, bringing fresh spring water to public fountains, baths and a few privileged private customers. The Romans weren't the first civilization to have a fresh water supply, but their engineering skills set the gold standard for the rest of the world to follow.

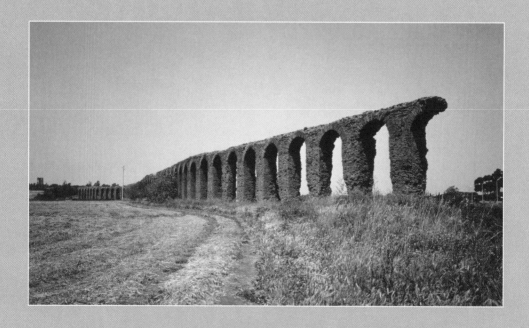

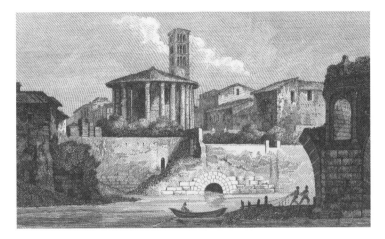

Outfall of Rome's Cloaca Maxima ("Greatest Sewer") as it drains into the Tiber River. Today it still carries rainwater from the city center to the river, running beneath the ancient forum and emerging by the Ponte Rotto.

THE CLOACA MAXIMA

The people of the later Indus Valley Civilization (ca. 2600–1900 BCE) understood the importance of not contaminating their water supplies, and they emptied and cleaned their cesspits regularly. The Minoans of 2000 to 1500 BCE used underground clay pipes to bring them fresh water, and had flush toilets to dispose of waste. In ancient China, officials regularly inspected the waterways and removed all animal and human corpses to prevent disease. However, the ancient Romans were among the first in the world to construct what could properly be called a sewage system: the Cloaca Maxima, which was built about 600 BCE to drain local marshes and carry effluent into the Tiber River via underground channels.

The main sewer was a covered canal, and separate branches served the main public buildings, such as the Baths of Diocletian, as well as the city's palaces. Private houses would have a cesspit into which residents emptied their chamber pots through a hole under the staircase—although it was not uncommon for them to be emptied out of windows onto unwary passersby. Fullers used urine for laundering clothes and provided urinals in which the public could donate supplies. The sewers were well maintained to clear blockages (which often occurred when citizens threw corpses into them) and parts of the Cloaca Maxima are still in use today. Sewer systems were adopted throughout the Roman Empire and the remains of one can still be seen in York, England.

> *The extraordinary greatness of the Roman Empire manifests itself above all in three things: the aqueducts, the paved roads and the construction of drains.*
> —**DIONYSIUS OF HALICARNASSUS,** *ROMAN ANTIQUITIES*, **FIRST CENTURY BCE**

SUPPLYING ROME WITH DRINKING WATER

For 441 years after the founding of the city of Rome, its people drank water from local springs, shallow wells and the Tiber River. However, as the population grew, the river and groundwater became heavily polluted as a result of citizens' cesspits leaking into them. Censors Gaius Plautius and Appius Claudius Caecus commissioned engineers to build the Aqua Appia to bring freshwater from a source in central Italy. It entered the city in the east, flowed through catch basins where the sediment settled, then was taken via lead pipes into the city center. Only a few private households had their own supply, but several tried to steal water by slipping a branch pipe into the main supply, a process known as "punching."

Water ran continuously through the public latrines, baths, and fountains, then wastewater flowed into the sewer. Huge tanks of water were used to stage sham naval battles to entertain the crowds, and stores of water were also kept to combat the ever-present risk of fire breaking out. The Aqua Appia was the first of nine aqueducts built to supply freshwater to the city between 312 BCE and 50 CE, and it was noticed that outbreaks of diarrheal diseases, such as cholera, dysentery and typhoid, were significantly reduced. The water quality in Rome is still renowned for its freshness to the present day.

Lead Poisoning

Lead pipes (*fistulae*) were used to transport water from aqueducts into the center of Rome, and scholars once theorized that lead poisoning might have affected so much of the population that it became one of the causes of the downfall of the Roman Empire. More recent studies have shown, however, that the high calcium content of the water coated the pipes, preventing the absorption of lead. Besides, instead of being stopped by valves, the water flowed continuously, which would also have prevented lead uptake. There is no mass evidence of lead poisoning in the Roman skeletons dug up by archaeologists.

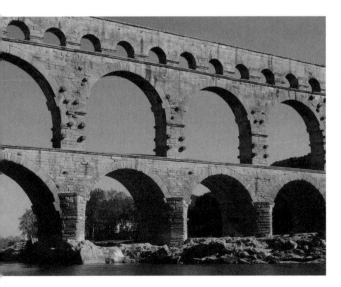

The Pont du Gard aqueduct was built in the first century CE to carry water from a spring through the foothills of the Massif Central, to the Roman colony based at Nîmes, in what is today southwest France.

THE ROMAN LEGACY

The Romans were way ahead of their times, but after the fall of the empire, the engineering skills they had used to build aqueducts were largely forgotten. It was only in the 17th century that cities throughout Europe began to devise ways of providing clean drinking water for their people. The New River was constructed between 1609 and 1613 to bring freshwater to the City of London from Hertfordshire, and thereafter many private companies established their own waterworks to supply other areas of the city. In 1842 New York became the first American city to tap a water supply outside its boundaries, bringing freshwater from the Croton River in Westchester County via an aqueduct, and other big cities followed suit—but there was still no prohibition on sewage being discharged into the water that citizens would drink.

During the 19th century, systems were devised for treating water by passing it through sand filters to remove suspended particles. In England a Public Health Act of 1848 and a Sanitary Act of 1866 made local authorities responsible for sewage disposal and the provision of a clean water supply, and other countries followed as it came to be understood that cholera and typhoid were transmitted in polluted water. In the early 20th century, purification of water with calcium hypochlorite became standard, and fluoride was added in many places to prevent tooth decay. New systems of treating sewage were also devised, with sewage plants using chemicals, sedimentation, and aerobic microorganisms to break down waste products.

A man covering his face to avoid inhaling miasma. Foul air was blamed for outbreaks of diseases, such as plague, cholera and malaria.

Miasma Theory

Many ancient cultures believed that epidemics of disease came from poisonous vapors, or "miasma," in the air, caused by rotting organic matter and poor hygiene. The Indians chewed paan leaves to counter the effects of miasma, and the Roman architect Vitruvius, writing in the first century BCE, wrote of the morning breeze bringing "the poisonous breath of creatures of the marshes." Romans believed that malaria (see pages 86–90) was caused by the bad air (hence its name, *mal'aria*), and this theory appeared justified when the incidence of the disease declined markedly after the building of the Cloaca Maxima. It was not understood that the draining of the marshes where mosquitoes had bred was the key factor. Miasma theory remained popular right up to the 19th century, when foul air from the Thames, the main river that runs through London, was initially blamed for cholera outbreaks in the city (see pages 106–109).

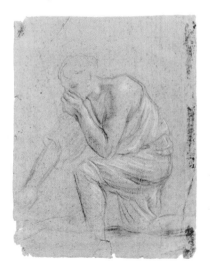

Dioscorides' *Materia Medica*

LOCATION:	Rome
DATE:	ca. 50–70 CE
FIELD:	Pharmacology

Pedanius Dioscorides was Greek but worked as a physician for the Roman army, which meant he traveled extensively and was able to examine plants from all over the empire. His extraordinary five-volume work entitled *Materia Medica* contains descriptions of more than a thousand herbal remedies with 4,740 different medicinal uses. By contrast, *The Hippocratic Corpus* included only 130 remedies. Dioscorides' research was so methodical and scientifically valuable that his work was quickly translated into other languages and remained the foremost reference right up to the 16th century.

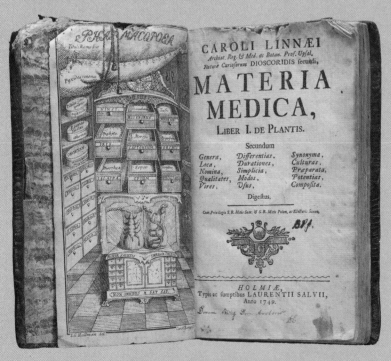

THE MIND OF A SCIENTIST

Many of the physicians in ancient Rome were of Greek origin and the system of medicine they followed came from the school of Hippocrates. Until 200 CE, anyone could declare themselves to be a physician, so there were a lot of charlatans who had received scant training. Roman naturalist Pliny the Elder complained: "There is no doubt that all these [physicians], in their hunt for popularity by means of some novelty, do not hesitate to buy it with our lives." However, Dioscorides had a scientific approach; he did not take anything for granted but personally tested every medicine he listed in his herbal compendium, over the course of his long career.

Entries are organized according to their medicinal uses, for example warming, binding, softening, cooling and so forth. For each he gives the plant's names and synonyms; its habitat; medical uses and how to prepare and administer the drugs; its effects and any cautions; other uses of the plant; and how to detect counterfeit versions (he warns, for example, that valeriana is often adulterated with butcher's broom, which makes it hard to break and gives it an unpleasant smell).

No other herbal cornucopia gave such detailed and authoritative advice. New versions of the *Materia Medica* were produced, with commentaries by later authors. It is unclear whether the original had the careful illustrations that enhanced later ones, but Dioscorides' work remained the classic text. It is reckoned that about one fifth of the remedies he recommended would have had therapeutic benefits for his patients, and many are still used in one form or another.

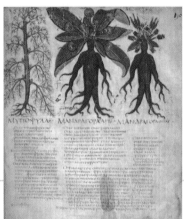

Dioscorides' illustration of and text on mandrake. Its root had soporific qualities, leading to its use as a surgical anesthetic and was also hallucinogenic and said to cause madness in large doses, whereas its juice was applied externally to relieve rheumatism.

Some of Dioscorides' Remedies

- **For sharpening eyesight and calming the nerves:** Vipers' flesh toasted with salt, honey, figs and nardostachys (spikenard) and made into a soup.
- **For gout:** A decoction of willow bark. Its active ingredient, salicylic acid, would be the key component in aspirin, developed in the late 19th century (see pages 138–41).
- **As an anesthetic for use during amputations or other surgery:** Mandragora (or mandrake) root. It contains hyoscyamine, a substance used for anesthesia in the early 19th century, before the introduction of ether (see pages 98–101).
- **As a pain-killer:** Opium, although Dioscorides warns that, when used to excess, it may cause lethargy and even death.

Galen's Phlebotome

LOCATION:	Greece and Rome
DATE:	ca. 150–210 CE
FIELD:	Anatomy, physiology, pathology, pharmacology, neurology

Galen studied medicine for 12 years, first at the Asklepeion (temple of Asklepios) in his hometown of Pergamon (in present-day Turkey) and then at various other places, including the famous school at Alexandria in Egypt, before setting up in practice. During his long career, he published prolifically and gave public lectures and dissections at which he expressed his strident views on medicine. Among the techniques he popularized was bloodletting, using a lancet known as a *phlebotome* to open the patient's veins. Some of his views were advanced for their time, whereas others were misleading, but his version of medicine would largely be accepted as fact until the 17th century.

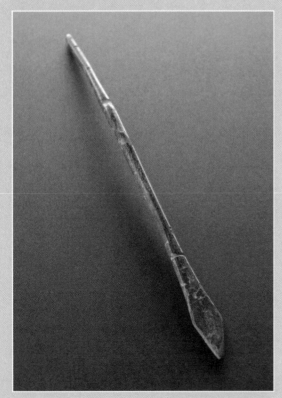

> *Employment is Nature's physician, and is essential to human happiness …. Laziness breeds humors of the blood.*
> —GALEN

PHYSICIAN TO GLADIATORS

When Galen returned from his medical studies abroad, he gained employment as a physician treating the gladiators at the arena in Pergamon and was soon acclaimed for his work there. Although 60 fighters had died under his predecessor, only five perished in his care. Galen used the huge gashes he treated in his patients as "windows" through which he could examine the veins, arteries, tendons and nerves—an invaluable opportunity at a time when human dissection was forbidden, and one that helped him to develop many of the theories with which his name would become associated.

In the 160s CE Galen moved to Rome, where he quickly made his name by treating the philosopher Eudemus, who recommended him to senators of his acquaintance. Before long, Galen was physician to Emperor Marcus Aurelius. He began performing live experiments and dissections on animals, mainly pigs and primates, and using them to promote himself and his writings. He gained a reputation for being cantankerous and does not appear to have had many friends in Rome, but everyone wanted to be treated by him simply because his cures were more effective than those of his contemporaries.

GALEN'S THEORIES

Galen accepted the Hippocratic model of human physiology but developed it through his own research.

Whereas his predecessors had believed that muscles were controlled by the heart, he demonstrated that the brain controlled the movements of muscles through the action of nerves. In one demonstration with a live pig, he cut through nerves one by one as the pig squealed in pain, and showed that only when he cut the nerve to the larynx did the squealing cease.

It had previously been thought that veins carried blood and arteries carried air or *pneuma* (see page 45), but Galen demonstrated that bright blood flowed in arteries and darker blood in veins. He believed that venous blood was continually being produced in the liver, and arterial blood

The Plague of Galen

Between 165 and 180 CE there was an outbreak in Rome of a particularly nasty plague that had a mortality rate of 7 to 10 percent. Galen traveled back to his hometown, no doubt anxious to avoid infection, but he was recalled by Marcus Aurelius, who wanted him to help in treating it. In his writings Galen describes the symptoms as fever, fetid breath, ulceration of the larynx and trachea, cough, catarrh, vomiting and skin eruptions that appeared on the ninth day of the illness. If the rough, scaly rash covering the body turned black, Galen predicted the patient would survive, whereas if they had black stools, he records that they generally died. Scholars now think it was probably smallpox (see pages 92–95) brought back from the Near East by soldiers. That outbreak killed an estimated five million people across Europe, including the Roman emperors Lucius Verus and Marcus Aurelius.

originated in the heart. He also believed in the theory of the four humors, and took it further to relate each humor to a personality trait. Those with an abundance of blood were of sanguine temperament and were extrovert and sociable; black bile produced a melancholic type who was creative and kind; yellow bile produced a choleric type who had energy and charisma; and phlegm produced a phlegmatic type who was affectionate and dependable.

A 15th-century miniature depicting Galen (seen on the left) instructing his assistant on the preparation of remedies using a mortar and pestle, while a scribe takes down his every word.

Galen showed that urine was formed in the kidneys and not the bladder, as had been previously thought.

He wrote dozens of medical texts in his lifetime, amounting to more than two million words, and his views were accepted as sacrosanct. They even became part of Church dogma in the centuries after his death, which meant that those who disagreed were afraid to speak up.

BLOODLETTING, THEORY AND PRACTICE

Galen valued bloodletting above any other therapeutic measure as a means of rebalancing the four humors and removing stale blood that had stagnated in the extremities, causing illness. It was prescribed for dozens of diseases from acne to pneumonia, epilepsy to stroke. He developed a complex system that laid down how much blood to remove, based on a patient's age, his constitution, the season, the weather and several other phenomena. He decided that different veins should be opened for different diseases: for example, a vein in the right hand would be opened to treat liver problems, the left hand would be used for problems with the spleen and one in the right elbow would be opened to stop a nosebleed from the right nostril. Fevers were relieved by letting copious amounts of blood—although Galen did warn about the dangers of cutting certain arteries, from which blood would spurt uncontrollably.

Galen had many followers in his advocacy of bloodletting; it was recommended in many later Indian and Islamic medical texts. Some religions advised bloodletting on saints' days, and the Jewish Talmud earmarked four days in particular on which it should be carried out, whereas other faiths aligned bloodletting sites with the positions of the stars.

> *[Galen is] first among doctors and unique among philosophers.*
> —EMPEROR MARCUS AURELIUS,
> AS REPORTED BY GALEN HIMSELF

Phlebotomy (cutting the vein) was the original method favored by Galen for bloodletting, but new methods that came into use over the centuries included scarification, cupping and leeches. (Cupping is a technique, sometimes used in preparation for bloodletting, in which heated vessels are applied to the skin, creating a vacuum which stimulates blood flow.)

Even after William Harvey had demonstrated the circulation of the blood in 1628 (see pages 72–75), disproving the theory behind bloodletting, it continued to be carried out in barbershops. When President George Washington caught a throat infection, he asked to be bled—and died after almost half his blood was removed over the course of 10 hours. There was no evidence of the technique being effective, but the belief that it cleared out weak or infected blood was hard to give up. Bloodletting was recommended in a medical textbook as recently as 1923. There are a few instances—but only a few—in which it could have been effective. It would have temporarily relieved high blood pressure, it could help to relieve fluid buildup in congestive heart failure and it might have had sedative effects for very agitated patients. In all cases, however, it would weaken the patient and reduce their likelihood of recovery.

How Much Blood?

Galen was the first physician to calculate how much blood should be let, and he recommended that 1.5 pounds (680 g) was the most and 7 ounces (200 grams) the least that would be effective. Avicenna (see pages 52–55), writing in the 10th century, calculated there were 25 pounds (11.3 kg) of blood in a man and that he could lose 20 pounds (9 kg) without dying. Today, we know that an adult weighing 150 pounds (68 kg) has 9 or 10 pounds (4–4.5 kg) of blood and that if he or she loses 10 percent or more, there will be a sudden drop in blood pressure, which will normally rise again within around 30 minutes. If more than 40 percent is lost, however, the patient probably won't survive unless the blood is immediately replaced by transfusion.

A surgeon prepares to open a vein in his patient's forearm while a boy holds a bowl to catch the blood. Bloodletting was the recommended treatment for virtually all ailments, including hemorrhages.

The Hôtel-Dieu

LOCATION: Paris, France
DATE: 651 CE
FIELD: Medicine, surgery

As soon as human beings began to settle in large communities, there was a need for institutions to care for the poor and sick. The wealthy were treated in their own homes, but the poor who had the misfortune to become ill would otherwise be left to lie in the streets. Religions that preached charity as a key virtue became responsible for running early hospitals, from the Greek *Asklepeion* to the Islamic *bimaristan* and the hospices of Christian military orders. The Hôtel-Dieu in Paris, France, is the oldest hospital in the world that is still open today, and its history gives an insight into the development of hospitals through the ages from charitable guesthouses to centers for medical research.

> *It may seem a strange principle to enunciate as the very first requirement in a Hospital that it should do the sick no harm.*
>
> —FLORENCE NIGHTINGALE,
> *NOTES ON NURSING,* 1859

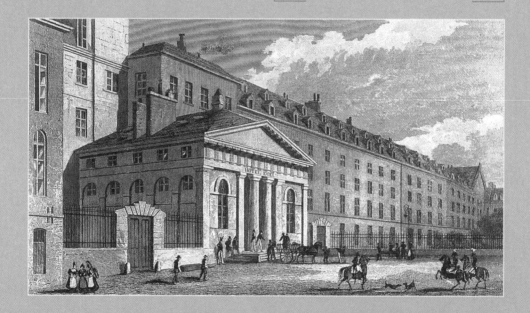

EARLY HOSPITALS

The Greek *Asklepeia*, built to honor Asklepios, god of healing, are the first recorded institutions where the sick came to be diagnosed and treated. In the Asklepeion of Epidaurus, three surviving marbles dated 350 BCE note the case histories of 70 patients who were treated there for ailments, including abdominal abscesses and foreign bodies that required removal. In India the *Charaka Samhita* of 150–100 BCE mentions houses for dispensing charity and medicine, and the Roman Empire had *valetudinaria* for treating wounded soldiers, gladiators and slaves. By the late 300s CE, Christian missionaries, such as the Order of St. John, were building hospices along their pilgrimage routes to care for the poor and needy, but their remit was focused on feeding and clothing widows and orphans and offering hospitality to strangers rather than attempting to cure the sick.

The First Council of Nicaea in 325 CE ruled that a hospital should be built in every cathedral city, and among the first cities to comply were Constantinople and Caesarea in modern-day Turkey. It was 651 CE when St. Landry, the Bishop of Paris, founded his city's first hospital, the Hôtel-Dieu, overlooking the Seine River, on the Île de la Cité. It was funded by the city's wealthy folk, but in the early years it did little more than feed and shelter the poor and infirm; there was no expectation that the sick might be cured and sent back into society.

THE HÔTEL-DIEU

In medieval times, Paris's Hôtel-Dieu was an immensely overcrowded place of last resort for the poor and sick, where little in the way of medical care was offered. In 1580 a new rule instructed that physicians had to visit patients twice a week, but there were often as many as 3,500 patients huddled within the hospital walls, and as many as six sharing each bed. Those with leprosy and tuberculosis were accommodated alongside the mentally ill, making it an unhealthy

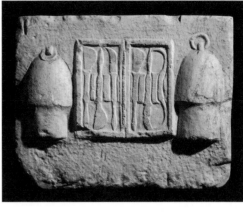

Relief on the Asklepeion of Athens, which was built after 420 BCE on the southern slope of the Acropolis. A place of rest for pilgrims, it also offered medical treatments.

Islamic Hospitals

There is an obligation in Islam to look after the sick, regardless of their background, religion or ability to pay for care. Institutions known as *bimaristan* opened in Damascus and Baghdad in the eighth century, offering a range of medical and surgical treatments. They took a much wider range of patients than those admitted to early Christian hospitals, also caring for the elderly, the mentally ill and those convalescing from illness. Bimaristan were not religious institutions but employed Christians and Jews as well as Muslims, and their services were generally free, although individual physicians might charge. By the 10th and 11th centuries, some bimaristan had their own pharmacies and outpatient departments, and employed both male and female staff.

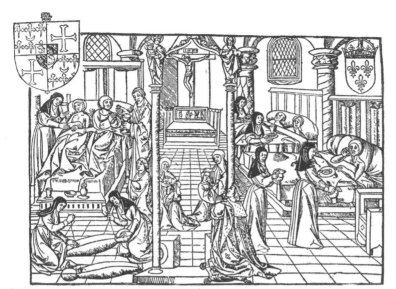

A ward in the Hôtel-Dieu, showing nuns attending to patients. In the left foreground they are sewing the dead into sheets. The hôtel was subsidized by noble families who hoped to earn their place in Heaven.

and uncomfortable place to be. By the 18th century, there were eight physicians and a hundred surgeons employed there.

In 1772 the Hôtel-Dieu had to be rebuilt following a catastrophic fire. During the French Revolution, several new hospitals were created in Paris and they began to specialize, with separate ones for the mentally ill, for those with venereal disease, for children and for geriatrics. The death rate was higher in the Hôtel-Dieu than at other hospitals, but that was largely because it admitted most of the victims of serious accidents that occurred in the city center.

It was rebuilt again in the mid-19th century and is still a busy working hospital for Parisians today. In a reflection of the hospital's origins as a charitable refuge, it retains the name Hôtel-Dieu, meaning "House of God."

FROM RELIGION TO SCIENCE

During the Middle Ages, monks and nuns ran the majority of European hospitals, and they were usually funded by the nobility, who made generous endowments in the hope of earning their spiritual reward in heaven. These nobles did not like to see their money wasted, so there was often

Leper Colonies

Leprosy is mentioned in an Egyptian papyrus of ca. 4000 BCE, and it spread through Europe after the return of Alexander the Great's troops from the East in the 320s BCE. The disease caused physical disfigurement and disability, and it was commonly thought to be the result of a curse or a punishment by God, so lepers were shunned. In medieval times, they had to ring a bell as they walked outdoors to let others avoid them, and they might also have had to wear special clothing. Leper colonies, known as *leprosaria* or lazar houses, were established in remote places or on islands, where lepers could be quarantined. In 1873 Dr. Gerhard Hansen of Norway discovered the bacterium that causes leprosy, and the first medicine to treat it successfully was developed in 1941. Europe's last leper colony, on the Greek island of Spinalonga, closed only in 1952.

an attempt to distinguish the "deserving" from the "undeserving" poor when deciding who got treatment. The Protestant Reformers of the 16th and 17th centuries rejected the idea that you could buy a place in the hereafter, and in Protestant countries hospitals became secular institutions funded by the Crown or the municipality, although private benefactors, or subscribers, were still important.

Hospitals gradually became places for the sick instead of the poor; the latter went to workhouses. The mentally ill went to special asylums, and those with physical ailments stayed in general hospitals. Wards often specialized in particular types of ailment, and in large hospitals facilities were made available for surgeons to do research. In 1859 the English nurse and reformer Florence Nightingale helped to establish professional training for nurses (see pages 110–13), which fundamentally changed the day-to-day running and efficiency of hospitals.

Still, hospitals remained dangerous places to be in the 19th century and the well-to-do preferred to be treated in their own homes, even having surgery at home rather than mingle with the underclasses. It was only in the 20th century that expensive new technology, such as x-ray machines, meant the wealthy had to go to the hospital to receive state-of-the-art treatment.

> *A hospital is, of all social institutions, the one in which perhaps the greatest mixture of motives, the most incompatible ambitions and the most vexatious vested interests are thrown together.*
> —**JOHN LANGDON-DAVIES,**
> *WESTMINSTER HOSPITAL: TWO CENTURIES OF VOLUNTARY SERVICE, 1952*

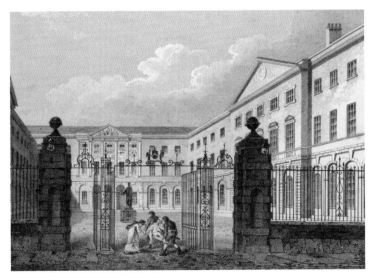

Guy's Hospital, London, was founded in 1721 by bookseller Thomas Guy, with money he had made investing in the South Sea Company. Originally used to accommodate patients who were deemed incurable, it is today a major teaching and research center.

Ten Treatises on the Eye

LOCATION:	Baghdad, Iraq
DATE:	Ninth century CE
FIELD:	Ophthalmology

It was a mystery that taxed cosmologists as much as it did scientists and physicians: How did images of the outside world make their way through the eyes to the brain, where we could perceive them? Hunayn ibn Ishaq, influential author of *Ten Treatises on the Eye*, proposed that they traveled from the object through the air to the back of the eye, where they mingled with aqueous humor, which then flowed through tubes to the brain. He may have been wrong about that aspect, but his book was the first to explain the anatomy of the eye systematically, and it represented a significant leap forward in the understanding of ophthalmology.

I pray that God may keep you and hope that you and others ... should benefit from the book for many years to come, and that my reward should be your good wishes.

—HUNAYN IBN ISHAQ,
TEN TREATISES ON THE EYE

EARLY APPROACHES

Eye diseases were prevalent in the ancient world, but the struggle to understand the causes and devise the best methods of treatment were fogged with misinformation and religious dogma. Writing in 2250 BCE, Hammurabi (see pages 16–17) described a physician opening an abscess in a man's eye with a bronze knife—a risky procedure because if the man had lost his eye, then the physician would have had his own eye taken out. The Ebers Papyrus of 1550 BCE (see page 15) devoted eight columns to eye diseases and herbal treatments for them, including onions, castor oil and pomegranate juice. The sixth-century BCE *Sushruta Samhita* (see page 18) described 76 diseases of the eye and gave the first written account of cataract surgery, in which a sharp needle was used to nudge the cataract to one side. Hippocrates' approach to treating eye infections was to draw humors away from the area by bloodletting and cupping at another site, then to apply "the milk of women and the gall of goats" as an ointment. Ophthalmology was somewhat looked down upon in Galen's time, but in the Islamic world of the ninth century CE, it attracted a lot of attention from scholars, and *kahhal* (oculists) were honored members of the royal household.

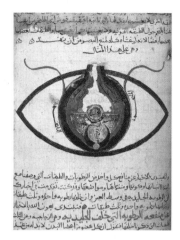

Illustration in the Cheshm Manuscript *(see page 46), ca. 1200 CE, showing pneuma flowing into the eye and mingling with the aqueous humor. The manuscript was discovered in a Persian library.*

Caliph Harun al-Rashid founded a House of Wisdom in Baghdad in the ninth century, with the aim of translating the works of Greek, Latin and Indian scholars into Arabic and promoting research among Islamic intellectuals. Hunayn ibn Ishaq learned about medicine in Baghdad, then traveled overseas to perfect his language skills, and on his return it is said that he could recite the works of Galen by heart. Fluent in Arabic, Syriac, Greek and Persian, he promoted a new style of translation that rewrote the original to make it read well for its new audience. He was placed in charge of the House of Wisdom, in which role he wrote 36 books of his own, 21 of them on medicine, as well as translating the works of others. He was particularly renowned for his translations of Plato, Aristotle and Galen, as well as the Old Testament (he worked from the Greek text known as the Septuagint).

Cosmological Pathways

Pneuma was the ancient Greek word for "breath," but it also meant "spirit" or "soul" or "life force." Pneuma was believed to travel through the arteries from the heart to the brain, where it produced thought. Hunayn ibn Ishaq's theory of vision, derived from Galen's, was that this pneuma traveled through the air back to the eye before flowing to the brain in the aqueous humor. He described how if one eye was closed, the visual pneuma was redirected to the other, causing the pupil to enlarge. Aristotle and Hippocrates had also believed that fluid was the medium by which images of the outside world were received by the brain, and Aristotle speculated that three tubes behind the eyes met within the skull.

THE *TEN TREATISES ON THE EYE*

In his masterwork, *Ten Treatises on the Eye*, Hunayn ibn Ishaq described the spherical shape of the lens, the sclera (outer covering of the eyeball), veins and arteries, the retina, the cornea (transparent covering of the iris and pupil) and the uvea (pigmented layer), opining that each of them was arranged in cosmological harmony. He said that sight was the highest of the five senses, corresponding to the element of fire, which is composed of a flame, red heat, and light. His detailed description inspired a famous illustration of the eye (shown on page 45) in the *Cheshm Manuscript* about 1200 CE.

Many other Islamic physicians wrote books on the eye, each taking knowledge a little further. Ali ibn Isa, writing in ca. 1010 CE, produced *The Notebook of the Oculists*, containing descriptions of more than 100 eye diseases; it went on to become the textbook most widely referred to by later ophthalmologists. Ammar bin Ali al-Mawsili wrote the *Book of Choices in the Treatment of Eye Diseases*, which describes six case histories in which he treated cataracts with his own invention: a fine hollow needle inserted into the eye, through which soft cataracts could be sucked out. It was an extremely successful operation, and one that in modified form is still used today. In the 13th century Ibn al-Nafis wrote *The Polished Book on Experimental Ophthalmology*, with one section on theory and another explaining the preparation of medicines for use in the treatment of eye complaints.

Cataract surgery in medieval Europe: A knife was inserted through the cornea to force the cataract out of its capsule and down to the bottom of the eye.

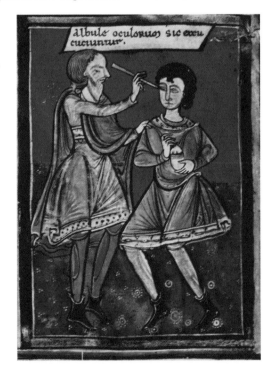

albule oculorum sic excuruntur.

INTO THE FUTURE

Many early civilizations developed their own versions of goggles to protect the eyes from harsh light, but English friar Roger Bacon was the first to describe, in his 1268 *Opus Majus*, the way that a plain convex lens with a thickness of less than its radius would magnify text when rested on a page. Alexander de Spina (d. 1313), a Dominican monk based in Pisa, may have been the person who first developed a method of balancing lenses in front of the eyes, thereby creating the world's earliest eyeglasses. Their value was not fully appreciated at the time, because so few people could read, but they were invaluable to monks who spent their days translating and transcribing manuscripts.

Leonardo da Vinci (see page 63) made the discovery that the retina, not the lens, was the organ of vision, and he explained how the eye works by means of a camera obscura—a darkened box or chamber fitted with a pinhole or lens through which light enters and projects an inverted image on the opposite wall. In 1851 Hermann Ludwig Ferdinand von Helmholtz invented the ophthalmoscope, enabling physicians to see right to the back of the eye, to the optic nerve—the real connection between eye and brain that those early pioneers had been searching for without success.

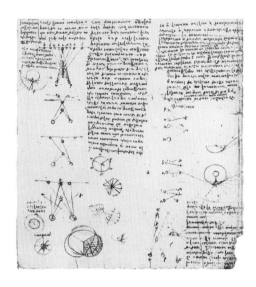

In his Notebooks, Leonardo da Vinci explained how light rays traveling from an object to the eye were refracted and an inverted image was focused onto the retina. He dissected many eyes but was unable to explain how images reached the brain.

Regulating the Profession

The medieval world of medicine was awash with charlatans, and ophthalmology was no exception. In the Ottoman Empire, itinerant eye surgeons known as "sons of the swallow" operated on cataract patients using a knife and had a poor success rate—which possibly explains why they were itinerant. In the Islamic world, physicians were examined on Hunayn ibn Ishaq's *Ten Treatises on the Eye* and forbidden to perform eye surgery if they could not demonstrate that they understood anatomy as described therein. An inspector known as a *muhtasib* could arrive unannounced to observe operations and impose penalties for low professional standards. Penalties ranged from beating on the soles of the feet to a warning of divine punishment on the Day of Resurrection. (He also inspected shops, and there are stories of cooks being boiled alive in their own cooking pots for selling putrid meat, and bakers being thrown into their furnaces for selling poisonous corn products.)

The School of Salerno

LOCATION: Salerno, Italy
DATE: 10th century
FIELD: Anatomy, surgery, pharmacology

If thou to health and vigor wouldst attain, Shun weighty cares—all anger deem profane, From heavy suppers and much wine abstain.
—JOHN OF MILAN (ATTRIBUTED)
REGIMEN SANITATIS SALERNITANUM, CA. 12TH–13TH CENTURIES

Salerno became the world's first true medical school in the 10th century simply because it happened to be in the right location at the right time. In the southern part of the Italian peninsula, the medical learning of the Greek, Roman, and Arabic lands came together, brought by travelers and Crusaders who stopped off en route to the Near East, and their texts were translated by scribes at the adjoining Benedictine monastery of Monte Cassino. Patients came to recuperate in the mild climate, followed by physicians who hoped to treat them, and the school that developed in Salerno became so famous that in 1224 it was decreed the only place in the world where the qualification of "doctor" could be obtained.

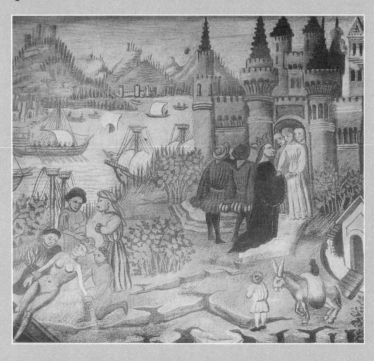

FOUR SCHOOLS OF THOUGHT

During the Dark Ages physicians in Europe were trained in monastic hospitals, where they undertook apprenticeships and studied texts transcribed by monks; but the Church was eager that there should be no practicing for financial gain, and limited the procedures they could carry out. The Benedictines had a more liberal tradition than most, and the monastery of Monte Cassino had both a dispensary and a well-stocked library. The medical school did not exist as an actual institution until the 13th century, but a group of four scholars are credited with beginning a system of teaching in Salerno back in the 10th century: a Jewish rabbi called Elinus, a Greek called Pontus, an Arab called Adale and a native of the town, who may have been a monk called Alphanus. This could be a legend, but it reflects the multicultural atmosphere that made Salerno such a unique place for physicians to study.

We know that an 11th-century merchant called Constantinus Africanus became ill while in Salerno and was not impressed when the physician who came to treat him did not even ask for a urine sample. He sailed home to Carthage, where he studied medicine for 3 years and collected many medical books, then he brought them over to Salerno where, with his knowledge of Greek, Latin, and Arabic, he was able to help translate them at the monastery. These works included many important Arabic texts that had not been seen in Europe before and formed a significant contribution to the Salerno library.

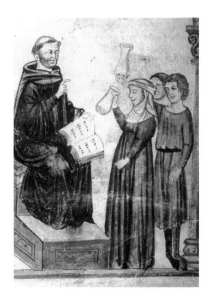

Constantinus Africanus examines a patient's urine. The use of urine to diagnose ailments goes back more than 6,000 years to the earliest civilizations. At first it was inspected visually, but during the Middle Ages, Paracelsus and others began to use distillation techniques.

Regimen Sanitatis Salernitanum

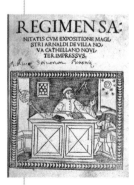

The title of this influential textbook translates as *Code of Health of the School of Salernum*. It contains 842 lines of verse advice on food and drink, motion and rest, sleeping and waking, air and dreams, as well as medical matters. It is said to have been written for Robert, Duke of Normandy, the eldest son of William the Conqueror, who spent the winter of 1096 in Salerno and later returned there for treatment of an infected arm wound. Its authorship is uncertain, but modern scholars think it may have been composed by John of Milan, who was head of the Salerno school. Although it was intended for the layperson, it became a key text for trainee physicians and was copied into several languages for use at schools elsewhere.

STUDYING AT SALERNO

As word of Salerno's fame spread, students came from across Europe to study there. They learned the works of Hippocrates and Galen, Aristotle and Avicenna, free of Church supervision. Lessons included anatomy, bloodletting, dietetics, medicines and surgery. They also learned how to conduct themselves as physicians when taking histories and examining patients, and the rules of patient–doctor conduct. Medicinal plants were grown in the school's garden and apothecaries visited to instruct students on the preparation of drugs. Once they passed the first set of examinations, they were awarded the title *Magister* (Master), which meant they were allowed to teach, but they had to study to a higher level to achieve the title Doctor.

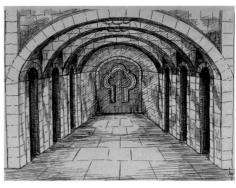

The crypt of the teaching hospital at Salerno. Greek was the spoken language used at the school but texts were in both Latin and Greek.

Famous pupils included a 12th-century female physician known as Trota of Salerno, to whom several influential books on women's health are attributed: *Book on the Conditions of Women*, *On Treatments for Women* and *On Women's Cosmetics*. She specialized in obstetrics and gynecology, and topics covered in her books include methods of restoring virginity and how to repair lips cracked from too much kissing.

> *Either the man or the woman may be "at fault": The woman may be too thin or too fat, or her womb may be so slippery that the man's seed cannot be retained. The man's seed, in turn, may itself be too thin and liquid, or his testicles may be so cold that he cannot generate seed.*
>
> —TROTA OF SALERNO, *CONDITIONS OF WOMEN*, 12TH CENTURY

Medieval Women in Medicine

Salerno was unique in letting women study medicine. Across the rest of Europe they could practice as midwives or what were known as "wise women," but would find themselves in trouble if they advertised themselves as physicians. Once it became illegal to practice medicine without a university degree, and universities stopped accepting female students, women were excluded from most branches of medicine. In Paris in 1322, five women went on trial charged with practicing medicine without a licence, and although one of them produced eight patients who testified that she had cured them when male doctors had failed, they were all found guilty and excommunicated.

Roger of Parma, who graduated from Salerno in the early 13th century, wrote *Chirurgia*, a much-admired book on surgery, in 1180. He advises using wet dressings on wounds, explains how to rebreak bones to correct poorly healed fractures and describes the use of ligatures if a hemorrhage could not be stopped with cauterization or styptics (substances that prevent bleeding). Roger went on to become the chancellor of the medical school at Montpellier in the south of France, and is often referred to as the founder of surgery.

REGULATING THE STUDY OF MEDICINE

In the 12th century Robert, King of the Two Sicilies, decreed that all doctors had to complete preliminary studies followed by 4 years of medicine at a university as the minimum requirement for a medical degree. In 1224 his grandson, the Holy Roman Emperor Frederick II, ruled that "no one could practice medicine unless they were examined before the faculty of Salern." He added that they needed to be at least 21 years old and to have studied for at least 7 years.

Similar laws passed across Europe led to the establishment of other medical schools: at Paris and Montpellier in France; Parma, Padua, Bologna and Ferrara in the Italian peninsula; and Tübingen in what is now Germany. Courses took an average of 4 or 5 years. Salerno's remained the most prestigious degree throughout the 12th and 13th centuries, but after the town was sacked by the Holy Roman Emperor Henry VI in 1194, the Montpellier School began to take precedence. All the same, the Salerno School continued until it was closed by the French Emperor Napoleon in the early 19th century.

Barber-Surgeons

Many physicians refused to perform surgery—in fact, in many places they weren't allowed to—and this role was taken over by barber-surgeons, who trained as apprentices in a craft guild instead of at a medical school. They could extract teeth, set fractures, and let blood as well as cut hair and sell medicines. Operations that required abdominal incisions were performed for only life-threatening conditions or those that were excruciatingly painful, such as bladder stones. Barber-surgeons sometimes advertised their services by hanging a bucket of blood and a bloodstained rag outside their shops, and this developed into the red-and-white striped pole that is still seen today. Surgeons were addressed as "Mr." instead of "Dr."—a practice still used in Great Britain to this day.

A traditional red-and-white barbers' pole in Edinburgh, Scotland. In the United States, the poles commonly have red, white, and blue stripes.

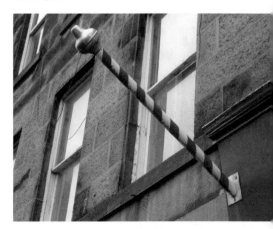

Avicenna's Tomb

LOCATION:	Hamadan, Iran
DATE:	1037 CE
FIELD:	Surgery, pathology, pharmacology

The great Persian has still a large practice, as his tomb is much visited by pilgrims among whom cures are said to be not uncommon.
—CANADIAN PHYSICIAN
DR. WILLIAM OSLER, 1913

During what is described as the Golden Age of Islam, from the eighth to the 13th centuries, when the caliphates of the Persian peninsula (loosely speaking, present-day Iran) subsidized research and learning, many great thinkers emerged, but perhaps the greatest of them all was Ibn Sina, known in the West as Avicenna. He wrote on philosophy and mathematics, poetry, astronomy, geography and psychology, but he is best known today for his *Canon of Medicine*, a five-volume work containing a million words. It soon became the standard medical textbook used in universities throughout Europe, and in the Arabic-speaking world Avicenna replaced Galen as the foremost medical eminence.

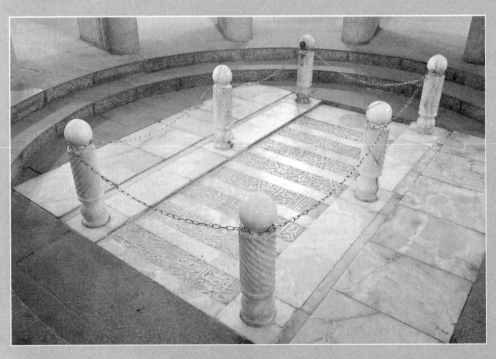

THE GOLDEN AGE

There were many pioneering medical scientists in the Arabic world around this period. Muhammad al-Razi was a physician of the ninth to 10th centuries who taught at the *bimaristan* in Baghdad and at Rey near Tehran, and who wrote more than 200 medical treatises, many of them very prescient. He gave accurate descriptions of measles and smallpox (see pages 92–95) for the first time in medical literature, and he proposed that fever might protect the body from disease. Avicenna, born 11 years after the death of al-Razi, would be scathing of his predecessor, saying that he "should have stuck to testing stools and urine," but his writings were significant at the time.

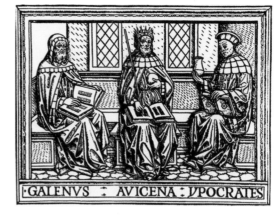

Three great teachers of medicine: Galen, Avicenna and Hippocrates in an image at Avicenna's tomb in Hamadan, Iran. They lived centuries apart but shared many beliefs on treating disease.

What we know about Avicenna's life mainly comes from the autobiography he dictated to a long-term student of his. He tells us that he was a child prodigy who could recite the entire Koran by the age of 10, and by 18 was a respected physician. He successfully treated an emir of the Samanid dynasty and in return was delighted to be allowed access to the royal library, which contained the works of Aristotle, Galen and Hippocrates. He wrote his first book at the age of 21 and went on to write 450 works, 150 of them on philosophy and 40 on medicine. The volatile political landscape forced him to travel for much of his adult life, but he settled for a while in Isfahan in Persia, where he held a Friday court at which scholars debated philosophical issues.

Avicenna was a hardworking physician, teacher and author, but he also found the time and energy for attending parties, where he was known for his love of lively music, strong drink and promiscuous womanizing. When his contemporaries suggested he take better care of himself, he replied, "I prefer a short life with width to a narrow one with length."

Aristotle

Aristotle was one of the most influential philosophers and scientists of the fourth century BCE, best known for his works on biology. He had been a student of Plato, but after his teacher's death he adopted scientific and empirical methods of testing his theses that displeased the religious authorities of the day but would appeal to Avicenna 14 centuries later. He described four qualities—hot, cold, wet and dry—that would later be applied to humoral theory. He suggested that tuberculosis was an infectious disease, an idea rejected by Hippocrates but accepted by Avicenna. Whenever Galen's anatomical theories were at odds with those of Aristotle, Avicenna sided with Aristotle, and through his writings he was influential in the rehabilitation of his illustrious predecessor.

THE *CANON OF MEDICINE*

Avicenna was not a humble man and he wrote his *Canon* fully intending it to be an all-encompassing work that would teach medicine as a complete, integrated subject. It took him 8 years, from 1015 to 1023, and achieved his aim of becoming a bible of medicine that supplanted Galen in the Arabic world; it was used as a set text in European universities at least until the 17th century. There are 5 volumes:

The meal should include: (1) meat especially kid of goats, veal and year-old lambs; (2) wheat, which is cleared of extraneous matter and gathered during a healthy harvest without ever being exposed to injurious influences; (3) sweets (fruits) of appropriate temperament.

—AVICENNA, *CANON OF MEDICINE*, 1015–23

- Volume 1: Anatomy, physiology, definitions of health and illness, the causes and treatments of disease
- Volume 2: The first definition of a scientific method of testing new drugs, with seven key rules, some of which are the basis of clinical trials today
- Volume 3: The pathology of 21 separate organs and systems in the body, from head to toe
- Volume 4: Fever, crisis and diseases that affect many parts of the body simultaneously; diagnosing symptoms and forming prognoses; minor surgery
- Volume 5: A manual for the preparation of pharmacological compounds, listing 760 drugs, with their method of application and effectiveness

Information was arranged logically, and Avicenna made several conclusions that advanced contemporary thinking. He described cancer as a swelling or tumor that grew rapidly, often in hollow organs such as the lungs, then spread to other organs. If small cancers were caught early and excised, with the surrounding blood vessels cut off, he wrote that they could be cured, but in late-stage cancers he advised no treatments other than dietary. He described how certain illnesses could be spread by water, the soil or mosquito bites. He explained how to introduce an

Illustration on the back cover of Avicenna's Canon of Medicine *showing a physician taking a pulse. He thought the quality of the pulse was dependent on the interaction of the four humors.*

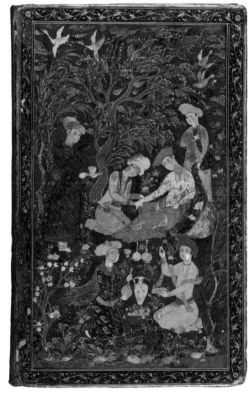

oropharyngeal tube (a device inserted into the throat to keep the airway open) to help those who are choking, and recommended that physicians use tracheotomy (cutting into the windpipe) only as a last resort. And he wrote that for good health, we should aim for a mixture of exercise, good food and adequate sleep.

AVICENNA'S LEGACY

The *Canon of Medicine* was written in Arabic but was quickly translated into a number of other languages, including Latin, German, French, Persian, Hebrew, Chinese and English. The *Canon* was printed in book form in 1472–73 and became one of the most popular medical texts. Its influence began to decline from the 16th century but it was still in use in the 18th century.

Avicenna died in 1037 in controversial circumstances. He succumbed to colic and treated himself with eight self-administered, celeryseed enemas in a day, along with mithridate, a mild form of opium. It may be that his servants mixed five measures of the active ingredient instead of two into his enemas, causing ulceration of the colon, or perhaps they got the dose of the opium wrong, but at any rate he died at the age of 57. A classic square mausoleum with domed roof was built for him at Hamadan in northwestern Persia, inscribed with verses from the Koran. In the mid-20th century, a grander mausoleum with a spindle-shape tower was built on top of the older memorial to mark the millennium of Avicenna's birth.

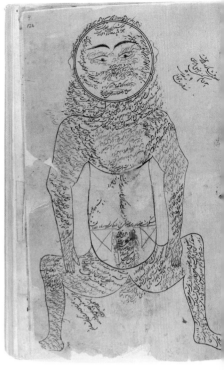

The muscular system, as shown in the Canon of Medicine. *Avicenna believed that regular massage, cold baths, exercise, sleep and food kept the body strong.*

Avicenna's Rules for Testing New Drugs

- **Experiments should be made on humans, not animals, for the most accurate results**
- **Drugs should be pure and not adulterated with any other substance**
- **They should be tested on simple instead of compound diseases**
- **They should be tested on two contrary diseases to test the effectiveness for each**
- **The potency of the drug should relate to the strength of the disease**
- **The time the drug takes to act must be observed**
- **The effect of the drug must be seen consistently for it to be declared a cure**

Plague Doctor's Mask

LOCATION:	Europe and Asia
DATE:	14th–17th centuries
FIELD:	Epidemiology, bacteriology

In 1346 a deadly disease arrived in Europe that would kill 60 percent of the population over the next 7 years and fundamentally change the medieval world view. King Philip VI of France blamed a conjunction of three planets, which caused "great pestilence in the air," and this so-called "miasma" was the most widely blamed cause. Others thought the plague was God's punishment for their sins and turned to faith healers for help. Many physicians refused to treat plague victims, but those who did adopted a macabre, birdlike mask in a futile bid to stop them from catching the disease.

The best of our popular physicians are the ones who do the least harm. But unfortunately some poison their patients with mercury, and others purge or bleed them to death ... there are others who care a great deal more for their own profit than the health of their patients.

—PARACELSUS, 1537

PLAGUE SYMPTOMS

The first symptom people with plague noticed was a painful bubo, or swelling, on the lymph nodes of the groin, armpit or neck, which oozed blood or pus if cut open. Next, the victim would experience acute fever and would vomit blood, which was followed by the appearance of frecklelike black or purple spots or a rash on the skin. This disease caused death in 80 percent of people. We now know it was bubonic plague, and the mortality rate, if untreated, remains the same in the 21st century as it was in 1346.

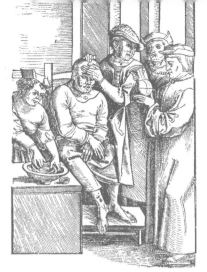

There were variations in the pattern of symptoms. Sometimes the infection traveled into the lungs, where it caused the person to cough up blood and experience respiratory problems. This variety, known as pneumonic plague, caused death in 90 to 95 percent of people and could be spread by sneezing. If the patient succumbed to septicemic plague, developing purple patches (*purpura*) on the skin, the death rate was more or less 100 percent. This form was spread by contact with open sores.

The 14th-century plague was called the Black Death because the characteristic buboes turned black, and black spots and boils might erupt all over the person's skin.

It wasn't discovered until the end of the 19th century that bubonic plague is caused by the *Yersinia pestis* bacterium, which blocks the digestive tract of fleas who catch it. The fleas get hungry and try to feed aggressively on their hosts, most commonly rodents. As the fleas regurgitate due to the blockage, the rodents are infected. After large numbers of the rodent hosts have died of the disease, the fleas move on to other hosts—human beings or domestic animals such as cats, dogs, oxen and donkeys—and the cycle continues. It can be passed from

Drawing of a flea seen under a microscope by Robert Hooke (see page 83), published in his Micrographia of 1665.

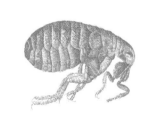

A Warm-Weather Disease

There were clues that could have helped medieval folk to understand the disease, had they known where to look. First of all, it was a disease of the warmer seasons, because the flea population died back in winter. In England, before the plague arrived, the highest mortality rates were in the winter months, when airborne contagious diseases were at their height, but after 1348 the greatest mortality was between July and September. When mapping plague outbreaks, they could have noted that it spread at about 25 miles (40 km) a day by ship or 1¼ miles (2 km) a day by road, and when an infected ship arrived in port, it took 23 days for the first plague death to occur in a human being, corresponding to the time it took the bacterium to kill native rodents then infect human hosts.

human to human but by far the most frequent method of infection was through a fleabite. Back in medieval times, people had no idea where the disease was coming from or how to combat it, and the lack of success their physicians had in treating it would lead to a loss of confidence in the profession as a whole.

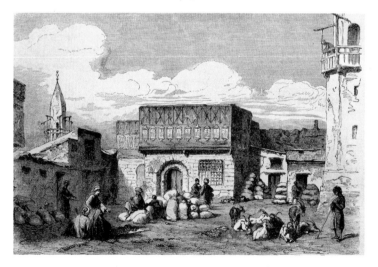

THE PLAGUE OF JUSTINIAN

The first recorded instance of bubonic plague occurred in 541–542 CE. The outbreak appears to have started in China and traveled to North Africa along trade routes, both overland and by sea. Citizens of the Roman Empire imported large quantities of grain from Egypt, and it was stored in huge vats that made perfect breeding grounds for rats. Soon plague broke out in Constantinople (present-day Istanbul, Turkey), and it was killing 5,000 a day at its height (10,000 according to Procopius, a contemporary historian). From there the disease moved into the Islamic territories and west into Europe.

Rattus rattus has long been blamed for the four centuries of plague in medieval Europe, but modern research suggests an Asian gerbil may also have carried Yersinia pestis, and that human-to-human transmission was possible.

The Roman emperor Justinian did not deal with the outbreak sympathetically. The prices of agricultural produce rose when farmers succumbed to disease, but he insisted his subjects must continue to pay taxes at the same rate to subsidize his great armies. He even ruled that if a man died, his neighbor must take over responsibility for his property and pay taxes on it as well as his own. According to Procopius, Justinian caught the plague himself but was among the lucky ones who recovered. Across Europe and Asia, 50 million would die between 541 and 750, and many historians credit the plague named after Justinian as instigating the decline and fall of the Roman Empire.

A market in Cairo, Egypt. In the 1340s, new and larger types of ships were plying trade routes, and many countries began to import agricultural produce instead of growing their own. But wherever the ships went, plague followed.

THE BLACK DEATH

In the late 1320s, plague broke out in Mongolia and spread west along trade routes to the Black Sea. From there it continued into southern Europe and the Middle East, reaching Alexandria in 1347, England in 1348, Norway in 1349 and Russia in 1351. Contemporary records describe dead bodies littering the streets and mass graves overflowing in cemeteries. It is estimated that Paris, France, lost half its population of 100,000, whereas Venice in Italy, and Hamburg and Bremen in Germany lost 60 percent of their citizens. The plague spread swiftly as people fled to avoid it and took the infection with them. The most terrifying aspect was that no one knew what caused it or how to avoid catching it.

King Philip VI of France asked a team at the University of Paris to investigate the causes, and they came up with the answer that the ill-favored conjunction of three planets was responsible, combined with earthquakes that released noxious poisons from the earth, and storms that spread those poisons. Desperate citizens sought someone to blame, so any wandering beggars, itinerant friars or pilgrims could find themselves under attack. Lepers (see page 42) came in for particular prejudice because it was thought the oozing sores in their skin could be plague-related. Others turned on Jews, Romanies and other foreigners who were thought to be carrying the disease and infecting others. In France and Germany, Jews were accused of causing plague by poisoning the wells, and despite calls by the Church to desist from attacks, 2,000 Jews were killed in Strasbourg in

Popular Remedies for the Black Death

Apothecaries sold all kinds of remedies to combat the plague. Antipestilence medicines varied from place to place but a popular one consisted of marigold flowers and roasted eggshells warmed in ale. Legend has it that four thieves in Marseille, France, who were caught robbing the dead offered to share their remedy for avoiding the plague in return for leniency. When the offer was accepted, they explained that they washed their skin with a herbal vinegar that came to be known as Marseille vinegar. Some swore by carrying nosegays or strong-smelling flowers to ward off "bad air," and there were numerous charms, spells and incantations that could be tried.

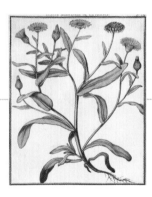

Dried flowers of the pot marigold (Calendula officinalis) were reputed to draw evil humors out of the head.

> *In 1374, a fanatical sect of dancers appeared in the Rhine, convinced that they could put an end to the epidemic by dancing for days and allowing other people to trample on their bodies …. By the time they reached Cologne they were 500 strong, dancing like demons, half-naked with flowers in their hair. Regarded as a menace by the authorities, these dancers macabre were threatened with excommunication.*
>
> —CATHARINE ARNOLD, *NECROPOLIS: LONDON AND ITS DEAD*, 2006

February 1349. More were burned in Basel, and the Jewish population was wiped out in Mainz and Cologne later that year. Ships arriving in Venice from infected ports were quarantined for 40 days (the Italian word *quarantina* means "a period of 40 days"). This measure, at least, may have helped to slow the spread of the disease.

> *Black or purple spots appeared on the arms or thighs or any other part of the body, sometimes a few large ones, sometimes many little ones. These spots were a certain sign of death.*
> —GIOVANNI BOCCACCIO, *THE DECAMERON*, 1348–53

PLAGUE DOCTORS

Towns were desperate to find physicians to treat their plague victims and were prepared to pay a premium for them. In 1348, the Italian city of Orvieto hired Matteo fu Angelo for the sum of 200 florins a year, which was four times the going rate. As well as treating the sick, plague doctors were charged with recording deaths, witnessing wills and, in some cases, trying to impart some ethical lessons—for example, admonishing those who abandoned family members in an effort to save themselves.

Some plague doctors were barber-surgeons, whereas others had no medical training at all, but that did not stop them from administering treatments. It was generally agreed that buboes should be lanced to release the humors and poultices applied to the wound. (In Justinian's day they had treated the wound site with boiling oil, which frequently finished the patient off immediately.) Alternatively, frogs and leeches were applied to the wound to release humors, or conventional bloodletting was used. Some advocated coating the victim in mercury and

Plague Doctor Costume

Plague doctors were understandably eager to avoid any contamination reaching their skin. In 1619 Charles de Lorme designed a costume consisting of a long waxed overcoat worn with boots and long gloves and topped with a birdlike mask with a beak shape at the front, which held straw scented with herbs and spices to filter out bad air. Ambergris, mint, camphor, cloves and lemon balm were popular choices. Plague doctors examined their patients with a cane instead of touching them directly. The costume was later adopted by the actors of the Commedia dell'Arte in Italy, and is still resurrected during the annual Venice carnival.

The mortality rate among plague doctors was high, because their macabre masks and costumes offered no protection from infection.

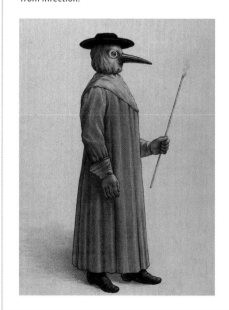

placing him in an oven, which must almost certainly have been fatal, and others used strong laxatives to purge the digestive system.

Not all "cures" were so radical. The 16th-century "prophet" Nostradamus (Michel de Nostredame) practiced as a plague doctor; he did not believe in bloodletting but recommended the more commonsense remedies of fresh air, clean water, a juice prepared from rose hips and the speedy removal of infected corpses. Swiss-German alchemist Paracelsus (Philip Bombast von Hohenheim) also worked as a plague doctor, and is said to have cured many people in the town of Sterzing by feeding them a pill made of bread and a tiny amount of their own feces.

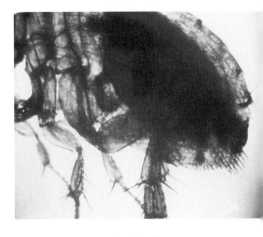

An oriental rat flea, Xenopsylla cheopis, containing a mass of Yersinia pestis bacteria. Worldwide, several thousand cases of plague continue to be diagnosed every year.

FROM THE 17TH TO THE 21ST CENTURIES

The Black Death of the 14th century remains the most devastating outbreak of plague the world has known. The infection never completely subsided and the 17th century saw some particularly deadly outbreaks. France and Italy lost a million people each in an epidemic that raged from 1628 to 1631, and the Great Plague of London in 1665 killed 100,000 people, one quarter of the population. What is known as the third bubonic plague pandemic hit China in the mid-19th century and the massive death toll included 10 million people in India alone. The first U.S. outbreak occurred in San Francisco in 1900–1904, and cases still crop up from time to time, particularly in the American West.

It was in Hong Kong in 1894 that Alexandre Yersin isolated the pathogen from the 1865 outbreak in China, which was named *Yersinia pestis* after him. In Karachi (in what is now Pakistan) in 1898, Paul-Louis Simond discovered that rat fleas were the primary vector of the disease and were being hosted by brown rats. By that stage, germ theory had supplanted miasma theory, and in the 20th century antibiotics would be produced to combat the plague. The reputation of the medical profession, which had failed to find a cure in 14th-century Europe, would take almost as long to recover.

> *The town growing so unhealthy, that a man cannot depend upon living two days*
> —SAMUEL PEPYS, *DIARY*, LONDON, 1665

De Humani Corporis Fabrica

LOCATION: Padua, Italy
DATE: 1543
FIELD: Anatomy

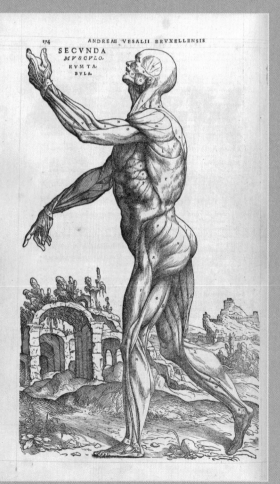

The prohibition on dissection of human beings had held back the study of anatomy for centuries, but with the spirit of scientific exploration that characterized the Renaissance it was once again permitted by ecclesiastical authorities, albeit in strictly limited circumstances. Galen's work was still viewed as sacrosanct in Europe and those who sought to criticize or correct him were treading on dangerous ground, but Padua University's Professor of Anatomy and Surgery, the Flemish-born Andreas Vesalius, was prepared to take the risk. Through public demonstrations of dissection, and his extraordinary illustrated books, he advanced the knowledge of human anatomy substantially.

> *Though you have a love for such things, you will perhaps be impeded by your stomach, and if this does not impede you, you will perhaps be impeded by your fear of living through the night hours in the company of quartered and flayed corpses fearful to behold.*
>
> —LEONARDO DA VINCI, NOTEBOOK, CA. 1510

THE FATE OF MURDERERS

In Alexandria, Egypt, in the 200s BCE, Ptolemy I Soter allowed the dissection of human bodies, especially those of criminals. Two figures, Herophilus and Erasistratus, made significant discoveries in the great medical school that arose there. Herophilus is seen by many as the founder of the science of anatomy, but his reputation was tarnished by claims that he performed live dissections on up to 600 prisoners. Later, Church prohibition prevented human dissection in Europe, and in the Islamic world it was considered taboo. This explains why Galen's dissections were all on animals. Buddhists in Tibet, however, practiced sky burial after ritual dissection of the dead, and their anatomical knowledge informed both Chinese and Indian medicine.

At the beginning of the 14th century, Mondino de Luzzi, a teacher at the University of Bologna in Italy, was given permission by the Vatican to perform the first public human dissections since Herophilus. According to contemporary descriptions, he sat on a high chair and explained proceedings to the audience while one of his junior assistants made the incision and another pointed out the structure in question. Mondino's book, the *Anathomia*, accepted Galen's views without question and is full of errors, but it paved the way for later anatomists.

Leonardo da Vinci dissected about 30 humans before he was ordered to stop by Pope Leo X. The 750 anatomical drawings he produced are, for the most part, remarkably accurate, but none of them were published in his lifetime because of his fear of censure. A few decades later, Andreas

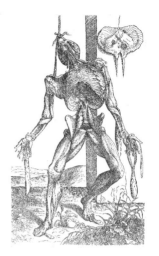

Dissection of a hanged criminal, pictured in Vesalius' 1543 book De Humani Corporis Fabrica, showing the source and position of muscles of the arms and legs.

A page from Da Vinci's Notebooks, showing the blood vessels of the abdomen. He famously used mirror writing, starting at the right side of the page and moving to the left.

Leonardo da Vinci

Artist, sculptor, engineer and quintessential Renaissance man, Leonardo da Vinci wanted to understand how the body was constructed. He performed his first dissection in 1506 on the body of a 100-year-old man whose peaceful death he had just witnessed. His drawings of human anatomy were ahead of their time, showing that the heart and not the liver was at the center of the blood system. He produced the first detailed drawings of the spine, and described cirrhosis of the liver and arteriosclerosis. He also invented new drawing techniques for showing cross sections and multiple angles. His papers were left to his heir, who made them available to several artists of the day, but had they been published at the time, they would have been a major contribution to anatomical research.

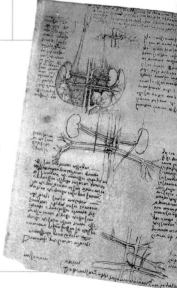

Vesalius was helped in his dissection research by a Paduan judge, who in 1539 ordered that the bodies of executed criminals should be made available to him, and the availability of the printing press (since about 1455) meant that Vesalius' discoveries could be quickly circulated around Europe.

DE HUMANI CORPORIS FABRICA

Cadavers could only be dissected in the 3 or 4 days following death, before the stench of decomposition became unbearable. Bodies decomposed more quickly in warm or wet weather, so the winter months were preferred for anatomical dissections. Andreas Vesalius liked to make the incisions himself, learning directly from observation instead of accepting the prevailing views, and that's what led him into direct conflict with Galen's model in several key areas:

Facing page: Vesalius instructed his printer that his drawings "have not been executed as simple outlines like ordinary diagrams in textbooks, but have been given proper pictorial quality."

Vesalius considered dissection to be useful for determining the best sites for bloodletting, and he encouraged doctors to make their own observations.

- Vesalius showed that the skeletal system was the framework of the body and examined the textures and strengths of different bones. He found that the sternum (or breastbone) was in three parts instead of the seven Galen had mooted, and that the lower jaw was one bone not two, but he explained that the disparities arose because Galen had worked on animals.
- He described the venous and arterial systems as "a tree whose trunks divide into branches and twigs" and listed more than 600 blood vessels. He did not believe Galen's claim of a porous membrane in the heart, but failed to find the "holes" that he proposed instead.
- He defined the brain and nervous system as the center of thought and emotion—not the heart, as Aristotle had thought—and showed that nerves originated in the brain and transmitted sensation to the muscles.
- He described the digestive and urinary systems, including the liver and gallbladder, and showed that the kidneys filtered blood as well as urine.

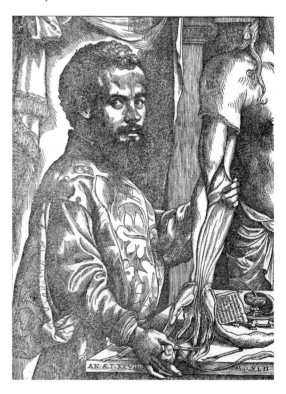

However, Vesalius was careful not to venture into territory that would upset the Church, so he came to no conclusions on the theory that the heart was the seat of the soul. All the same, critics were horrified at his contradictions of Galen, who was considered infallible. One suggested that the human body must have changed since Galen's time to account for the differences Vesalius was finding, because obviously the great Galen could not have been wrong.

BARBERS AND GRAVE ROBBERS

Vesalius was only 28 when his book *De Humani Corporis Fabrica* (*On the Structure of the Human Body*) was published, with 273 illustrations by artists from the school of Titian; He made sure of high production values by personally supervising the printing by the renowned Johannes Oporinus in Switzerland. Immediately the book was circulated around Europe to much acclaim. Vesalius was appointed physician at the court of the Holy Roman Emperor Charles V, but he was looked down upon by the other physicians, who mocked him for being a "barber." One of his enemies spread the story that he had performed a live dissection and had been forced as penance to make a pilgrimage to the Holy Land. He did, in fact, make a pilgrimage and died on the return journey, but the penance story has been disproved by scholars. All the same, it demonstrates the delicate ground on which Vesalius trod with his work.

> *Those who have dissected or inspected many [bodies] have at least learned to doubt, while others who are ignorant of anatomy and do not take the trouble to attend it are in no doubt at all.*
> —ITALIAN ANATOMIST GIOVANNI BATTISTA MORGAGNI, *LETTERS*, 1761

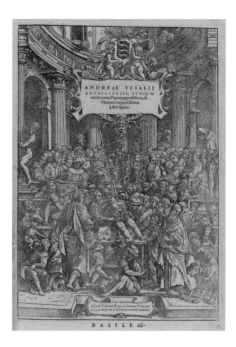

Autopsies

The study of human anatomy made it possible to see where disease had changed internal organs, and thus to establish the cause of death. A magistrate in Bologna, Italy, in 1302 requested a dissection to establish "fault" in a death he was investigating, and during the 15th century, the Florentine Antonio Benivieni carried out 15 legal autopsies. Giovanni Morgagni's 1761 book *On the Seats and Causes of Diseases* compared his observations of 700 different corpses, and in the early 19th century Carl von Rokitansky performed an average of two autopsies a day, 7 days a week, over 45 years, developing an approach that became generally accepted.

Throughout the 17th and 18th centuries, only certified anatomists could perform dissections, and then only in limited circumstances. The shortage of bodies led William Harvey (see pages 72–75) to dissect his own father and sister after their deaths, and there was a thriving market in dead bodies for dissection at medical schools. This led to the practice of grave robbing, and in Edinburgh, Scotland, in 1828 the notorious Burke and Hare murdered 16 people in order to sell their bodies for dissection. In the 21st century, computer modeling is replacing dissection as a method of teaching anatomy at some medical schools, although many argue that the hands-on method is best.

HUMAN ANATOMY IN RENAISSANCE ART

In the centuries before the Renaissance, the human body was seen as shameful and was only portrayed completely clothed, but the great cultural flowering that began in Florence in the 14th century led to a renewed interest in the sculptures of classical Greece, many of them nudes. The Greeks revered the body for its strength and beauty, and believed it was created in the image of the gods. As Renaissance artists turned once more to nude subjects, they had the new study of dissection to aid them and it became *de rigueur* for artists to view or even conduct their own dissections.

According to Renaissance chronicler Giorgio Vasari, Antonio Pollaiuolo was the "first master to skin many human bodies in order to investigate the muscles and understand the nude in a more modern way." His engraving *Battle of the Nude Men*, dating from 1465–75, emphasizes the muscularity of his figures. A number of artists produced studies of peeled-away skin and ripped-apart muscles, as if to prove they had attended a dissection.

The most famous Renaissance nude is unquestionably Michelangelo's *David*, the 17 foot (5.2 meter) tall marble figure he created between 1501 and 1504. Michelangelo had started dissection at the age of 18, after the prior of the monastery of Santo Spirito in Florence gave him access to bodies before burial,

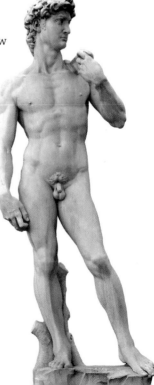

Michelangelo's David (1501–1504) demonstrates a clear understanding of the main muscle groups.

and this study shows in the anatomical accuracy of his sculptures. Scholars have pointed out just a few errors. The center of the *David*'s back is hollow instead of rounded, but Michelangelo explained that by saying that he lacked enough material in the marble block he was using. His head and hands, particularly his right hand, are unusually large, whereas the genitals are small, but this is part of the artist's vision of a man tensed in battle. The penis is uncircumcised, although David was Jewish.

THE ANATOMY LESSON OF DR. NICOLAES TULP

By the 17th century, public dissections in Protestant countries, such as Holland, had become social spectacles that the public could attend in return for a fee. Refreshments were served and the events were looked upon as fun excursions.

The Amsterdam surgeons' guild commissioned a portrait of their leading doctors every 5 years or so, and the young Rembrandt van Rijn was commissioned in 1632 to paint the dissection of an armed robber. Rembrandt changed the normal conventions of the genre by showing the corpse full-length in a Christ-like pose, with the doctors grouped around him. Their names are listed on the paper held by the man at the back. Dr. Nicolaes Tulp, the praelector of the Amsterdam Anatomy Guild, is showing the flexor muscles of the left arm, but he is not holding a cutting tool, because he would not have performed the dissection himself. The picture was universally praised for its accuracy, but, in fact, surgeons would invariably first open the chest cavity, before dissecting the limbs, because the internal organs would decay more rapidly than muscles. In 2006 Dutch researchers who restaged the scene using a real corpse found that there are some discrepancies in the layout of the tendons. In the corner of the picture is a textbook by Vesalius, the first master of anatomical illustration.

Rembrandt's The Anatomy Lesson of Dr. Nicolaes Tulp *(1632) features the corpse of Aris Kindt, an armed robber who had been executed by hanging that morning.*

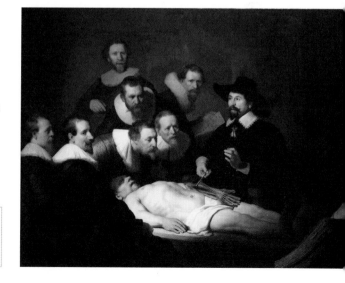

Choose only one master—Nature.
—REMBRANDT VAN RIJN

Santorio Santorio's Thermoscope

LOCATION:	Padua, Italy
DATE:	1612
FIELD:	Physiology

Although the humoral theory of Hippocrates and Galen was still adhered to by physicians in the late 16th and early 17th centuries, scientists were also beginning to apply empirical methods to the evaluation of disease and health. No one took the challenge quite as personally, however, as Santorio Santorio, who for 30 years weighed all the food and drink he consumed, and measured his excretions of urine and feces in an effort to understand the metabolism of the human body. He designed many pieces of equipment to further his research, but the one for which he is best remembered today is the thermoscope.

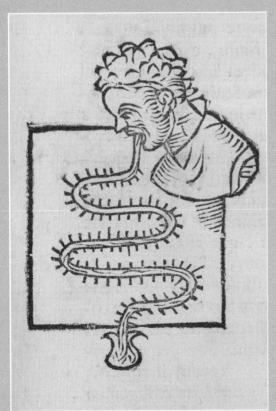

The patient grasps the bulb, or breathes upon it into a hood, or takes the bulb into his mouth, so that we can tell if the patient be better or worse, so as not to be led astray in knowledge of prognosis or cure.

—SANTORIO SANTORIO,
MEDICINA STATICA, 1614

A HISTORY OF FEVER

From antiquity, heat had been used as a method of curing all kinds of diseases from skin complaints through to dropsy. Hot water, steam baths and resting in ovenlike conditions were prescribed by cultures from American Indians to Chinese to ancient Egyptians. Hippocrates thought that heat drew forth corrupt humors, and said, "Give me the power to produce fever and I will cure all disease." Until Santorio, it was thought that the body temperature changed according to the temperature of the environment, and no one had the means to measure it.

In his work as Professor of Medical Theory at Padua, Santorio aimed to explain the workings of the body on mechanical grounds, and to that end he devised methods of measuring various phenomena, which he evaluated in huge statistical studies. He knew the great scientist, astronomer and inventor Galileo Galilei and his learned circle of friends from a period he had spent in Venice. Galileo had used his observations of the expansion and contraction of water and air at different temperatures to create a "thermoscope," in which bulbs of differing mass floated in a container of water. As the temperature of the water changed, some of the bulbs would sink while others remained afloat, and the number marked on the lowest bulb afloat gave the temperature of the water.

Santorio took Galileo's principle and applied it to a tube with a scale marked on it that could be inserted into a patient's mouth or held in his hand to take the temperature of the body. In this way,

Santorio's pulsilogium (below left) may be the first example in medical history of a machine devised to take physiological measurements. His thermometer (below right) was crude, but nonetheless revolutionary.

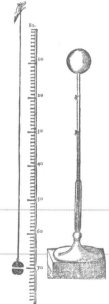

Santorio's Inventions

As well as improving on the thermoscope, Santorio also devised a gauge to measure wind speed, a meter to measure the strength of a current of water, an instrument for removing bladder stones, a trocar (piercing implement) for draining fluid from cavities and a *pulsilogium* to measure the pulse rate. Like his thermoscope, the pulsilogium was based on an invention of Galileo, who had constructed a small pendulum with the upper part attached to a scale. Galileo had shown that he could obtain a numerical estimate of the pulse by pressing the string until the oscillation of the pendulum coincided with the patient's pulse. Santorio created a more sensitive model with a lead bullet on the end of a cord and was able to measure slight differences in pulse rate that would have been otherwise undetectable, but no one at the time appreciated its usefulness.

he discovered for the first time that there is a normal range of human temperature. He didn't know how this knowledge could be applied to treating patients, but his contribution is no less significant for that.

ARS DE STATICA MEDICINA

Santorio spent most of his career amassing medical statistics, which he published in 1614 in a book entitled *Ars de Statica Medicina* (*The Art of Statistical Medicine*). It contained a record of his bodily functions over the previous 30 years. He had designed a weighing chair—basically a platform suspended from a moving arm—on which he weighed himself, his food and drink, and his excretions. Through it he found that for every 8 pounds (3.6 kg) of food intake, he excreted only 3 pounds (1.4 kg) of weight, and he explained the loss from the body as being by *perspiratio insensibilis* (imperceptible perspiration), following Galen's definition of respiration through the skin.

Perhaps Santorio's biggest influence on medicine was to apply the theories of physics, chemistry and mathematics to humans. He argued that the body was like a clock, made up of parts that worked together according to their size and position, a theory that moved away from Galen's view of qualities and essences. His work was not much appreciated at the time, and physicist Robert Boyle, writing in the 17th century, called the thermoscope "a work of needless curiosity, a superfluous diligence." It would take a couple more centuries before physicians completely appreciated the importance of measuring vital signs in the assessment of health and sickness.

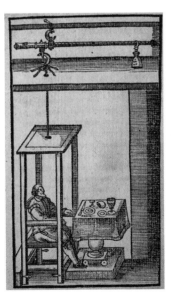

The weighing chair designed by Santorio. He devoted his life to quantitative experiments with the aim of explaining how the human body worked.

THE DEVELOPMENT OF THERMOMETERS

A number of 18th-century doctors—including Hermann Boerhaave of Leiden, Holland; Gerard Van Swieten, founder of the Viennese School; and Anton De Haen of The Hague, Holland—began to take the temperatures of their patients. They found that temperature was a useful way of charting the progress of disease, but few other physicians agreed. The thermometers of the day were huge, unwieldy objects that took a long time to get a reading, and it was 1867 before Thomas Clifford Albutt created a 6-inch (15-cm) thermometer that could take a temperature reading in 5 minutes.

The prevailing view remained that fever was a good thing, because it helped to heal disease, until Edinburgh physician William Cullen proposed in 1777 that fever was due to a suppression of the natural metabolism and that febrile patients should be cooled down. Cold baths, cool packs, even snow and ice were among the methods used before the development of medicines that could lower body temperature.

It was only in the 19th century that the association between infection and fever was recognized, when Carl Wunderlich published *The Temperature in Disease*, based on data from 25,000 patients, and introduced temperature charts.

In the 21st century taking temperature is standard procedure, and it is seen as one of the four vital signs alongside pulse, respiration rate and blood pressure. Normal temperature is 97.8 to 99°F (36.5 to 37.2°F) and fever is anything above 99°F (37.2°C), whereas below 95°F (35°C) is a sign of hypothermia.

> *The temperature may be determined with a nicety which is common to few other phenomena. The temperature can neither be feigned nor falsified. We may conclude the presence of some disturbance in the economy from the mere fact of altered temperature.*
>
> **—CARL WUNDERLICH,** *THE TEMPERATURE IN DISEASE,* **1871**

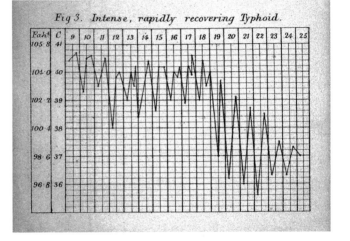

The temperature chart, introduced by Carl Wunderlich, medical director of the university hospital in Leipzig from 1850–71. His thermometer was 12 inches (30 cm) long and took 20 minutes to read a patient's temperature.

Harvey's Diagram of Blood Circulation

LOCATION: London, England
DATE: 1616–28
FIELD: Anatomy

[Harvey] had conducted himself so wonderfully well in the examination, and had shown such skill, memory and learning, that he had far surpassed even the great hopes which his examiners had formed of him.

—ITALIAN ANATOMIST
HIERONYMUS FABRICIUS, 1602

At the turn of the 17th century, theories on the cardiovascular system had advanced little since the work of Galen in Rome 1,400 years earlier. A few had tentatively tried to contradict Galen's findings but risked being accused of heresy; Spanish doctor Michael Servetus was burned at the stake in 1553 for his book *Christianismi Restitutio* (*The Restoration of Christianity*) in which he correctly described pulmonary circulation. Fifty years after that event, William Harvey began experiments and live animal dissections that would enable him to describe, for the first time, how the heart pumped blood in a circular route around the body; but he was understandably cautious about revealing his findings until he could back them up with solid empirical evidence.

FROM GALEN TO HARVEY

Until the 17th century, physicians believed there were two separate blood systems: the so-called "natural" system of venous blood, which was created in the liver and eliminated daily, and the "vital" system of arterial blood and spirits, which flowed from the heart, distributing heat and life. Galen taught that the arteries sucked in air and discharged vapors, and that the action of the lungs cooled the blood heated by the heart.

Arabic physician Ibn al-Nafis contradicted Galen in 1242, when he suggested that blood absorbed air in the lungs and carried it back to the right side of the heart before it was sent off around the body. Leonardo da Vinci made many sketches from his dissections of oxen and pigs, showing that the heart is a muscle with four chambers, and he showed that a pulse in the wrist could be created by contraction of the left ventricle. Sixteenth-century anatomist Jacques Dubois was the first to discover venous valves, but he could not explain them because he remained a firm believer in Galen's theories.

William Harvey (1578–1657) could draw upon the discoveries of all these men and more after an education that included study at the University of Padua under the famous anatomist Hieronymus Fabricius. Fabricius recognized that the valves in veins worked only one way, but was puzzled by their purpose. Fourteen years after graduating from Padua, Harvey would explain this in a lecture to the College of Physicians in London.

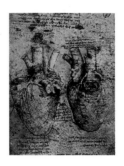

An illustration of the heart and its blood vessels by Leonardo da Vinci, ca. 1510. He was ahead of his time when he noted that eddies in the flow of blood caused heart valves to open and close.

DE MOTU CORDIS

In 1609 Harvey became Physician in Charge at St. Bartholomew's Hospital in London, and 6 years later he was appointed Lumleian lecturer to the College of Physicians. His role was to increase knowledge of anatomy, and he conducted a series of public dissections, many of them on live animals, during which he developed the groundbreaking theories he would announce to his fellows in 1616. It took a further 12 years before he published his lectures in 1628 in a book entitled *Exercitatio Anatomica de Motu Cordis et Sanguinis in Animalibus*, commonly known as *De Motu Cordis* (*On the Motion of the Heart*), complete with his detailed illustrations.

Witchcraft Trials

As a scientist who based his findings on experiment and evidence, Harvey was not a believer in witchcraft. He was asked to rule on the cases of four women suspected of being witches, and in each case he cleared them. He visited one of them, pretending to be a wizard, and asked to meet her "particular," whereupon she is said to have called a toad to drink from a saucer of milk. The woman left the room, and during her absence Harvey killed and dissected the toad; he found that it was not magical but a perfectly normal creature. The woman was at first angry when she returned to find her pet dead, until Harvey revealed the true purpose of his visit and the conclusion he had come to, upon which she must have been mightily relieved.

In his book he described the structure of the heart and demonstrated that the contraction of the left ventricle pumped blood to the arteries of the body, whereas the right ventricle pumped it into the pulmonary artery, the two acting in unison. He calculated that the heart beats 1,000 times every half hour and estimated that if the capacity of the heart was 1½ fluid ounces (43 ml) and it propelled ⅙ fluid ounce (4.7 ml) with each contraction, then it would require 540 pounds (245 kg) of blood a day—a volume that clearly could not be manufactured by the liver, as Galen had proposed. Repeated circulation of the same blood was the only plausible explanation.

Harvey tied ligatures around the arms of subjects and showed how the lower part of the limb became white from lack of arterial blood, while the veins swelled, and thus he demonstrated one of his key principles: that blood circulates around the body in one direction, with valves preventing it from flowing backward.

Harvey's findings were received with interest in England, where he was a much-respected figure, but with outrage in the rest of Europe. Not only did they contradict much of Galen's model, but they also questioned the usefulness of bloodletting, one of the key medical treatments at the time.

Facing page: Harvey demonstrating his theory of the circulation of blood to Charles I of England. The king, like his predecessor James I, had an eager interest in Harvey's research.

A 1647 woodcut showing a vivisection of a dog by Harvey, who believed dissections of living creatures were essential to demonstrate the circulation of blood. Between 1664 and 1668, 90 live dissections were reported to the Royal Society.

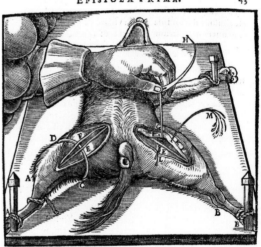

EPISTOLA PRIMA.   43

FIGURÆ EXPLICATIO.

A. *Crus canis dextrum.*   B. *Crus canis siniſtrum.*
C. D. *Ligatura ſubiecta arteriæ & venæ , qua femur firmiter conſtringitur , expreſſa in dextro crure, ne literarum linearumque confuſio in ſmiſtro crure ſpectatorem poſſet turbare.*
E. *Arteria cruralis.*   F. *Vena cruralis.*
G. *Filum quo conſtricta eſt vena & eſt elevata.*
H. *Acus, cui filum eſt traiectum.*
I. *Venæ pars ſuperior & detumeſcens.*
K. *Venæ pars inferior à ligatura intumeſcens.*
L. *Guttæ ſanguinis , quæ, éſuperiori parte venæ vulnerata , ſenſim diſtillant.*
M. *Rivulus ſanguinis, qui, inferiori venæ parte vulnerata, continuo exilit.*

F 2   vero

I have heard him say that after his booke on the Circulation of the Blood came out, that he fell mightily in his practise, and that 'twas believed by the Vulgar that he was crack-brained; and all the physitians were against his opinion, and envyed him.

—JOHN AUBREY, *BRIEF LIVES*, 1669–96

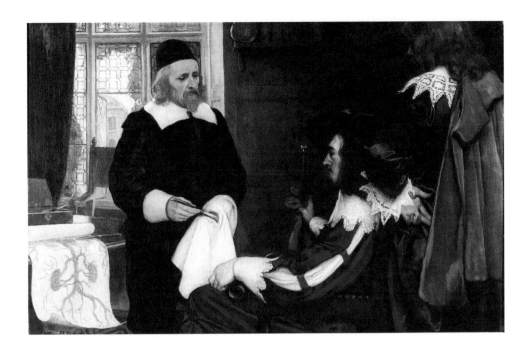

UNDERSTANDING EGGS

Harvey had a lot of criticism to contend with after publishing his masterwork, but it did not stop his research. In 1651 he published *On Animal Generation*, in which he was the first to suggest that the reproduction of mammals was caused by fertilization of an egg by a sperm, but he speculated that they were drawn to each other by some kind of magnetism. The true process would not be clear until microscopes came into use later in the century. He also demonstrated that an organism is not a preformed entity but develops gradually and is built up piece by piece.

Harvey retired from medical practice in 1645, but he had the gratification of knowing that his key discoveries had been accepted within his own lifetime. Still, the practice of bloodletting would continue for another two centuries, peaking in popularity between the 1830s and 1850s, when leeches were often used for the purpose.

Measuring Blood Pressure

Later, other scientists continued Harvey's work. In 1733, English clergyman Stephen Hales tried to measure the pressure that caused blood to flow by inserting an 11-foot (3.4-meter) glass tube into the artery of a horse. The amount by which the blood rose in the tube indicated the pressure in the artery, he surmised. In 1828 French scientist Jean Poiseuille used a U-shaped tube containing mercury to counterbalance the pressure of the blood, then in 1881 Austrian physician Samuel Siegfried von Basch designed the first sphygmomanometer—a device that could measure blood pressure without cutting open the patient. Blood pressure measurements went on to become a first-line test of the health of the cardiovascular system that Harvey had described so convincingly in the early 17th century.

Chamberlen's Forceps

LOCATION: London, England
DATE: Early 17th century
FIELD: Obstetrics

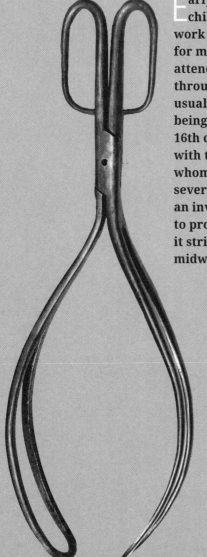

Early medical textbooks barely give childbirth a mention. It was women's work and the birthing chamber was no place for men. Midwives learned their trade by attending other women's deliveries and through their own experience, and skills were usually passed on by word of mouth instead of being written down in books. At the end of the 16th century, however, this began to change with the appearance of male midwives, of whom the Chamberlen family produced several generations. What's more, they used an invention that they claimed helped labor to proceed swiftly and safely, but they kept it strictly to themselves. No wonder female midwives were unimpressed.

And rather Dr. Chamberlane's work and the work belonging to midwifes are contrary one to the other for he deliv's none without the use of instruments by extraordinary violence in desperate occasions, which women never practised nor desyred for they have neither parts nor hands for that art.

—PETITION OF MIDWIVES TO COLLEGE OF PHYSICIANS, 1634

FROM ANTIQUITY TO THE MIDDLE AGES

There are records from 1500 BCE of herbal remedies for all kinds of issues of concern to women: contraception, infertility, pregnancy testing, abortion and speeding the progress of labor. In the second century CE, Soranus of Ephesus wrote at length about the qualities needed in a good midwife who, he said, should be responsible and literate, should love her work, and should be endowed with "long, slim fingers and short nails." Hippocrates wrote that a fetus could be aborted if the woman kicked her heels into her buttocks until the seed dropped out, and an early pregnancy test advised women to urinate on a bouquet of wheat, barley, dates and sand; if the grains sprouted, the woman was pregnant.

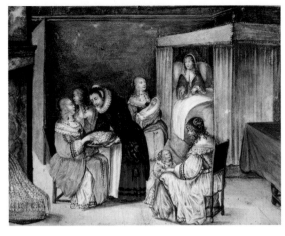

Pregnant women had to provide refreshments for the "gossips" who sat with them during labor.

The leaves of hemp were smoked or the seeds or oil used in cakes to produce analgesic and narcotic effects. Chinese herbalist Chen-Nung warned 5,000 years ago that "if taken in excess, [it] will produce hallucinations."

Traditionally, when a woman went into labor, along with friends and family, the other women in the neighborhood would come to sit with her, and it was her obligation to provide food and drinks for all. These women were her "sisters in God," a name which was shortened first to "God-sibs" and then "gossips." They would sit chattering and mopping

Folk Remedies for Delivery

An infusion of raspberry leaf was said to induce abortion in the early months of pregnancy, and to speed and ease delivery at term. In some areas, hawthorn was used for the same purpose. Cakes might be offered to the woman in labor (and her husband, too), containing hempseed and gin, along with rhubarb root and grated dandelion root. Henbane was used as a pain-killer, although it could produce hallucinations and even seizures and tachycardia (excessively rapid heartbeat). In ancient Egypt, fumigation with fat from a hyena was said to produce immediate delivery, and many midwives used oily substances scented with sweet-smelling herbs to massage the belly. In some parts of Scotland, a poultice of seaweed was traditionally applied to the belly to help expel the afterbirth.

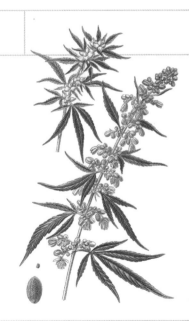

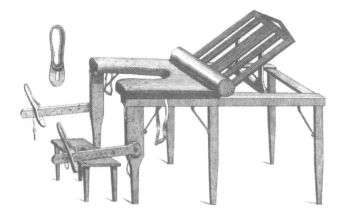

her brow throughout the hours of labor. The midwife might offer herbal remedies and would have scissors, linen and birthing stool at the ready.

The risks were high. During the Renaissance, women had between 1 and 2 percent chance of dying during each birth, so if they had a large family of 8 to 10 children, the odds increased accordingly. The child, meanwhile, had a 20 percent chance of dying before the age of 5, so big families were essential. There was no notion that hygiene was important, so many women succumbed to infection, and postpartum hemorrhage carried off many new mothers.

Cesarean sections were uncommon—unless it was to retrieve a baby once the mother was already dead or dying—so there was little recourse if the child got obstructed in the womb or birth canal.

THE SECRETIVE CHAMBERLENS

In 1576 Huguenot refugees William Chamberlen and his son Peter fled France and arrived in Southampton, where William had a second son whom he also called Peter. Peter the Elder and Peter the Younger became barber-surgeons but the elder brother broke the rules of the College of Barber-Surgeons by prescribing drugs and spent some time in London's Newgate prison. He was released after the intercession of the Lord Mayor of London and the Archbishop of Canterbury, because by now the family had friends in high places. Peter the Elder later became physician and midwife to Queen Anne, wife of King James I, and then to Henrietta Maria, wife of Charles I.

It's not clear exactly which Chamberlen invented the obstetric forceps that would become their

An 18th-century birthing chair, in which women gave birth in an upright position. An early example is seen in an Egyptian wall painting, ca. 1450 BCE, and it is regaining popularity today, because it can speed deliveries.

Dr. Peter Chamberlen (1601–83), son of Peter the Younger, attended Queen Henrietta Maria at the birth of the future King Charles II. Chamberlen's reputation traveled far and wide: the Czar of Russia tried, unsuccessfully, to poach him.

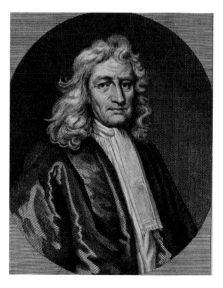

family's claim to fame, but they are thought to have existed long before Peter the Elder's death in 1631 and it is probable that he was the creator. Rickets was increasingly common in the 17th century and caused malformation of the pelvis, which meant more labors in which the baby became obstructed. The Chamberlens' device helped to pull the baby down the birth canal and was their attempt to help solve the problem.

From the start, the Chamberlens decided to keep their invention a family secret. When attending a woman in labor, two of them would arrive carrying a large box with gilded carvings. They would close the door to the rest of the household and, if the labor was proceeding slowly or the baby appeared to be stuck, they would blindfold the poor woman before bringing out their forceps. Those listening outside would hear ringing bells and a number of other peculiar noises, which made them think some kind of large machine had delivered the baby. No one ever saw them at work and, one way or another, the Chamberlens kept the secret of the forceps to themselves for more than 100 years.

THE SECRET IS OUT

In 1670 Hugh Chamberlen, eldest son of Peter the Younger, tried to sell the secret of the forceps to the French king's physician, François Mauriceau, for the sum of 10,000 crowns. He claimed it could deliver any baby within 15 minutes, but when Mauriceau set him the challenge of delivering the baby of a woman with dwarfism and a deformed pelvis, Chamberlen failed. The secret remained hidden, although Mauriceau referred to the forceps in a book he wrote. In 1693 Hugh Chamberlen formed a partnership with a Dutch surgeon, Hendrik van Roonhuisen, to sell the forceps at an inflated price, and managed to persuade the Dutch authorities that no one should obtain a licence to deliver babies without first

The Forceps

Peter the Elder's own forceps were found in 1813 under the floorboards of the house where he had lived. Made of metal, the blades were straight in profile but had a curve for grasping the infant's head. Each blade was separate, but the two were locked together by a pivot on one blade that fitted into a hole on the other. An earlier pair just had a hole through which a cord could be threaded to fasten the blades together. It was a simple design that hardly warranted the great secrecy.

Paul Chamberlen, second son of Peter the Younger, designed an "anodyne necklace," which he claimed would help women have a safe pregnancy and easy labor, and it would also ease teething in the child. It became a best seller, perhaps due more to the family reputation for innovation rather than any great efficacy.

The pain involved is of the following sort: as if, for example, someone would throw an olive pit into a small-mouthed oil flask, the pit is not naturally suited to be taken out when it is turned on its side. In this way, then, the birth of the embryo laterally presented is also a very painful experience for the woman; it just does not go out.
—HIPPOCRATES ON BREECH BIRTHS, FIFTH CENTURY BCE

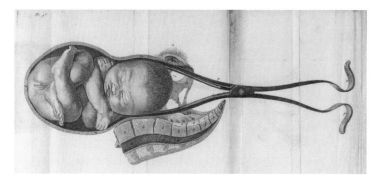

buying them. It was 1732 before a drawing of the forceps was published and they came into general use.

In 1747 French obstetrician André Levet modified the design of the original forceps to follow the pelvic curve so they could grip the heads of babies that were still high up in the pelvis. A Scotsman, William Smellie, developed his own style of forceps and taught many students to use them—an action that caused midwife Elizabeth Nihell to call him, indignantly, "a great horse-godmother of a he-midwife." As physicians increasingly moved into their territory, midwives were losing the tax-exempt state pensions they had previously been granted by local authorities, and they fought it all the way but to no avail. The men were in the birthing chamber, and they were there to stay.

Caricature of a man-mid-wife by Isaac Cruikshank (1793). Physicians were accused of demeaning themselves by doing "women's work."

DEVELOPMENTS IN THE 19TH AND 20TH CENTURIES

Childbirth was still an extremely dangerous process in the 18th century, with a mortality rate of around 25 women per 1,000 births. A number of developments over the next two centuries would bring that down:

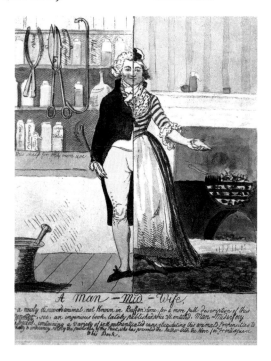

A Man — Mid — Wife

- From 1740 women started giving birth in lying-in hospitals, and by the 1790s one third to a half of all deliveries were attended by trained physicians. Midwives were still used, but in most countries they were forced to undergo training in order to be registered for practice.
- In 1818 London physician Dr. James Blundell carried out the first blood transfusion to treat hemorrhage after birth (see page 173).

- In 1842 obstetrician James Young Simpson suggested it might help to prevent infection if doctors washed their hands and disinfected their instruments between patients.
- In 1849 the same James Young Simpson developed an early kind of ventouse—a metal syringe attached to a rubber cup, to extract the baby by suction—but it was another century before it became popular, eventually being used more frequently than forceps.
- During the 19th century, ether and chloroform anesthetics (see pages 98–101) were used during childbirth.
- The introduction of antibiotics in the 1930s helped to combat deaths from puerperal fever and other infections.
- By the 1980s, ultrasound imaging (see pages 194–97) was becoming common. At first used only for high-risk pregnancies, it was soon available for all in the developed world.
- The world's first baby conceived by in vitro fertilization was born in 1978.

Other inventions, such as oxytoxic drugs to induce labor, episiotomies and safer cesarean sections also helped to reduce the level of deaths in childbirth. In 2013 the global figure for childbirth was 210 deaths per 100,000 live births, but the level was much lower in developed countries, with the lowest rate being only 3.9 per 100,000 in Italy.

Puerperal Fever

In 1797 the writer and women's rights campaigner Mary Wollstonecraft died from puerperal, or childbirth, fever—a bacterial infection of the female reproductive organs—10 days after the birth of her second daughter. There are descriptions of this type of fever in the writings of Hippocrates, but it wasn't until the mid-19th century that Hungarian physician Ignaz Semmelweis showed that it was contagious. One clinic in his hospital had a much higher rate of infection than another, and he realized it was because medical students were coming in from working on autopsies without washing their hands, and assisting the women giving birth. This was long before germ theory, and his findings were scorned and led to his dismissal. He later heard that physicians in England had started washing their hands and disinfecting instruments with chlorine 5 years earlier, and maternal death rates had plummeted as a result (see pages 128–31).

Prontosil, the first successful antibacterial medicine, came into use in 1935 and proved effective against previously life-threatening infections, including puerperal fever.

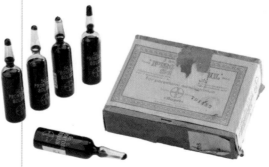

Van Leeuwenhoek's Microscope

LOCATION:	Holland
DATE:	1676
FIELD:	Bacteriology, protozoology

There was great alarm and no small degree of skepticism at England's Royal Academy in 1676 when they received a letter from Antonie van Leeuwenhoek saying that he had found tiny organisms, which he called "animalcules," swimming in a drop of water when viewed under his specially prepared lens. They commissioned physicist Robert Hooke to repeat the experiment and he found the same thing. Many of the mysteries of medicine were soon to be solved by these men, and others working both before and since, who learned how to see particles that were too small to be discerned by the naked eye.

> *In all falling rain, carried from gutters into water butts, animalcules are to be found; and in all kinds of water, standing in the open air, animalcules can occur. For these animalcules can be carried over by the wind, along with bits of dust floating in the air.*
>
> —ANTONIE VAN LEEUWENHOEK, 1702

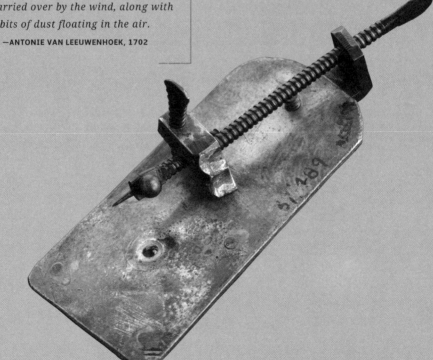

THE SECRETS UNDER THE LENS

Roger Bacon and others had created convex lenses that would magnify small letters for reading (see page 47). Taking their work a stage further, in 1595 Zacharias and Hans Jansen, Dutch makers of eyeglasses, put several lenses inside a tube and found that the magnification at the opposite end from the eye was greater than with one lens alone. They achieved a magnification of only ×9 and the image was somewhat blurred, but the principle of the compound microscope was established and others were curious to follow. Galileo Galilei made a compound microscope in 1625, calling it the *occhiolino*, or "little eye," but left it to others to use the technology on the human body.

In 1660 Marcello Malpighi examined human tissue under an early microscope and discovered the capillaries that William Harvey (see pages 72–75) had theorized about and failed to find; and in 1665 Robert Hooke published *Micrographia*, a stunning collection of illustrations showing what he could see through his own microscope (see page 57). Among his most important findings, he observed a structural mesh in a piece of cork, with cavities that reminded him of monks' cells in a monastery. He coined the name "cell" for these porelike structures.

Antonie van Leeuwenhoek (1632–1723) was an uneducated man, a draper by trade, who used magnifying glasses to check the thread counts of fabric. Grinding lenses was his hobby and it is estimated that he made and polished more than 550 of them with great perfectionism. He managed to make a single lens with a magnification of ×270—far greater than anything his contemporaries had achieved— and looking through it he came up with the revolutionary discovery that living things are made up of millions of tiny living parts that cannot be seen by the naked eye.

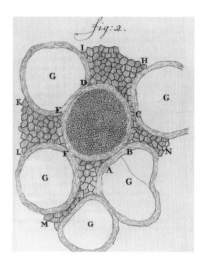

Van Leeuwenhoek's drawing of nerves in the spinal marrow of cows and sheep, published in his Epistolae Physiologicae, 1719. He was not university educated but was inspired in his research by Hooke's book Micrographia.

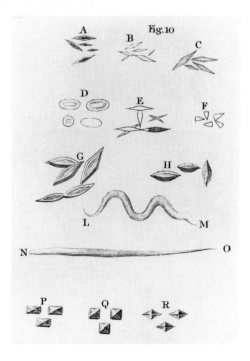

Microscopic animalcules discovered by Van Leeuwenhoek: "little animals ... very gently moving, with outstretched bodies and opened-out tails." These were the first bacteria ever observed.

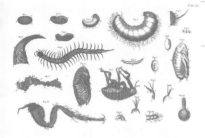

Refuting Spontaneous Generation

Spontaneous generation was the widely believed theory that living organisms could develop from nonliving ones, just as maggots appeared to do in a lump of meat. Van Leeuwenhoek showed this was not the case, demonstrating that weevils in granaries were grubs hatched from eggs that had been left there by winged insects, instead of creatures emerging from the wheat itself. He showed that fleas were not created from sand, as was thought, but that they reproduced just like other insects. He showed that shellfish came from spawn instead of the sand and mud of the seabed, and that eels were products of reproduction, and not made from the dew.

VAN LEEUWENHOEK'S FINDINGS

A friend introduced Van Leeuwenhoek to the Royal Society in England and he began writing to them about his discoveries. Between 1673 and 1723 he sent the Society a series of articulate and descriptive letters that it republished as reports.

In 1673 he wrote about his observations of the mouthparts of the bee, as well as the human louse and liver fluke. In 1676 he found tiny organisms in a drop of rainwater, and on further investigation he also found them in pond and well water and in the human mouth and stools. He drew the organisms in 1683, the first recorded images of bacteria. He also drew blood corpuscles, the striations in muscle tissue, nematode worms and crystals; but personally he considered his discovery of spermatozoa to be his most significant. He described not just human sperm but the sperm of mollusks, fish, amphibians, birds and mammals, and he concluded that fertilization occurred at the moment when the spermatozoon penetrated the egg.

Some of Van Leeuwenhoek's lenses were no bigger than a pinhead, and he mounted them between two brass plates that were riveted together, then focused, using screws. He was helped by his incredibly sharp eyesight and a dogged persistence that made him the first man in the world to view objects of a micrometer (one millionth of a meter, or 0.000039 inch) in size.

Spermatozoa of rabbit (figs. 1–4) and dog (figs. 5–8). William Harvey believed the egg contained everything needed for reproduction and many derided Van Leeuwenhoek's assertion that spermatozoa were essential too.

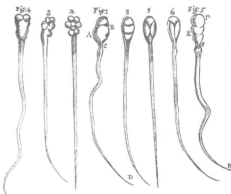

> *My work, which I have done for a long time, was not pursued in order to gain the*
> *praise I now enjoy, but chiefly from a craving after knowledge, which I notice resides*
> *in me more than in most other men. And therewithal, whenever I found out anything*
> *remarkable, I have thought it my duty to put down my discovery on paper,*
> *so that all ingenious people might be informed thereof.*
>
> —ANTONIE VAN LEEUWENHOEK, 1712

THE DEVELOPMENT OF MICROSCOPE TECHNOLOGY

A century after Van Leeuwenhoek, Carl Zeiss of Germany refined lenses in his microscopes to avoid optical defects, such as chromatic aberration, caused by different colors of light bending by different amounts as they passed through. Ernst Abbe, who worked for Zeiss's company, improved the quality of the lenses and achieved magnifications 10 times better than Van Leeuwenhoek had ever managed, allowing him to see objects of just 200 nanometers across (a nanometer is one billionth of a meter). It was impossible for optical microscopes to focus on objects that were smaller than the wavelength of light, so research stalled at that point for a few decades.

In 1899 a microscope was first used directly on the human body when Siegfried Czapski viewed the cornea through one, and in 1921, microsurgery was performed under a microscope—a technology that would continue to develop over the course of the next century and benefit millions (see page 199). In 1932 the first electron microscope was developed and a whole new world of magnification was made possible, with images several thousand times smaller than the wavelength of light becoming visible for the first time. By the end of World War II, a magnification of x200,000 was common, allowing researchers to make out the synapses between nerve cells, to identify viruses, such as the polio virus, and to see the granules that release histamines in mast cells.

Staining Cells

Staining is a technique used in microscopy to highlight cells of a particular type so their shapes and positions within larger structures can be viewed more clearly. Dyes are chosen that will be specifically taken up by particular materials. Common examples are carmine for glycogen, coomassie blue for proteins, crystal violet for cell walls, malachite green for spores and safranin yellow for collagen. Their colors can make cells look attractive, and a number of artists have been inspired by microscope imagery, but staining has also given the public the false idea that viruses are large, brightly colored organisms, whereas in fact they are colorless and smaller than the wavelength of light.

Stained electron micrograph, shown below right, of the 1918 influenza virus (see pages 152–53). The development of staining techniques allowed scientists to pinpoint individual structures in a way that was difficult in black and white.

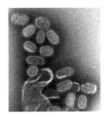 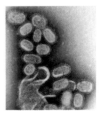

The Cinchona Tree

LOCATION: Ecuador
DATE: 1737
FIELD: Epidemiology, tropical diseases

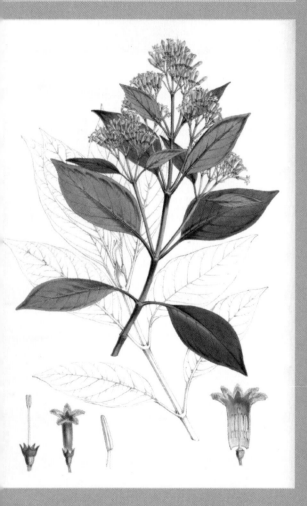

A disease causing severe fevers that subsided then recurred was described in Egypt, China and Greece as early as 2700 BCE. The Romans thought it was caused by bad air—*mala aria*—and knew it was more common in marshy regions. In Britain it was known as "marsh fever" or "tertian ague," the latter because the episodes of fever recurred every third day. In 1737 French explorer Charles Marie de la Condamine learned from native Ecuadorians that the bitter bark of the cinchona tree could cure malarial fever, but it would be another 150 years before anyone began to work out what caused it.

> *Sirius, harbinger of fevers,*
> *the evil star that dominates the*
> *night sky at harvest time.*
> —HOMER, *THE ILIAD*, CA. 760–710 BCE

CURE BEFORE CAUSE

No one knows the mortality rate for malaria before the 20th century, partly because it was often confused with other fever-producing diseases, such as typhoid, but we can be sure it was high. Some recent scholars estimate that around half of all the people who have ever lived were killed by malaria.

The *Huangchi Neijing* (see pages 22–25), written in China between 475 and 300 BCE, describes fevers accompanied by an enlarged spleen, and there are references to malaria-like illnesses in Chinese writings as far back as 2700 BCE. There is also mention of a herbal cure, the bitter juice of the artemisia plant, which is a key ingredient in one of the most successful malarial treatments of the 21st century.

Galen advised bleeding and fasting as a cure for malaria, whereas ancient Egyptians advocated consuming huge quantities of garlic. Avicenna recommended absinthe juice for a fever, whereas Dioscorides advised drinking absinthe for an enlarged liver but not while there was fever present. Southernwood and mugwort (both species of artemisia) were just two herbal remedies among hundreds of others, depending on the flora and fauna of the region.

A 1901 illustration of the lifecycle of the protozoan parasites that cause malaria. Sporozoites injected into the blood multiply in the liver, then invade the red blood cells, where they multiply again, causing fever at each multiplication stage.

Types of Malaria

At least four different types of malaria parasite infect human beings. Of these, *Plasmodium falciparum* causes the highest number of deaths worldwide, with complications including acute respiratory distress, encephalopathy and renal failure. In pregnant women it can cause miscarriage, stillbirth, and babies with low birth weight. *P. vivax*, *P. ovale* and *P. malariae* generally cause a milder form of malaria, but *P. vivax* and *P. ovale* can lie dormant in the liver and produce clinical symptoms years later. All cause the classic symptom of paroxysms, with a sudden feeling of coldness leading to shivering, then fever and sweating. In *P. vivax* and *P. ovale* the paroxysms recur every 2 days; in *P. malariae* they are every 3 days; and with *P. falciparum*, every 36 to 48 hours.

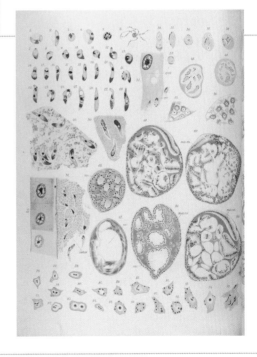

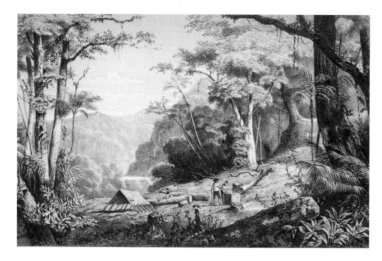

The Cinchona tree is native to Peru. During the harvest, bark is beaten off the branches, traditionally by women and children.

Malaria is believed to have been passed to man by gorillas back in prehistoric times, probably in Africa. European settlers would have introduced it to the Americas in the 16th century (along with a host of other diseases—see page 93). When Charles Marie de la Condamine went to South America to test Newton's theory that the Earth bulges at the Equator, he was told about the medicinal bark of the "fever tree," which was then unknown in Europe.

In 1880 at the Military Hospital at Constantine, I discovered, on the edges of the pigmented spherical bodies in the blood of a patient suffering from malaria, filiform elements resembling flagellae, which were moving very rapidly, displacing the neighboring red cells.
—CHARLES LOUIS ALPHONSE LAVERAN, 1889

He heard that the second Countess of Chinchón had been cured of malaria after bathing in a pool that was overlooked by fever trees. Condamine drew pictures of the tree, made copious notes and brought samples back to Europe. Soon everyone wanted some of this miracle bark. Charles II of England and the son of Louis XIV of France were both treated with it, and in 1742 the great Swedish botanist Carl Linnaeus named it *Cinchona*, after the countess it had cured.

THE SEARCH FOR THE CAUSE

Cinchona bark did not cure everyone, but it did appear to reduce fevers of the intermittent type. It is a muscle relaxant, so would have helped to ease the paroxysms that were part of the pattern of symptoms. Prevention would have been preferable, but for that it was necessary to understand the cause.

It had long been noticed that malaria was prevalent in swampy areas—in ancient Rome there had been repeated outbreaks because of the marshes that surrounded the capital.

Red blood cells being invaded by malaria parasites.

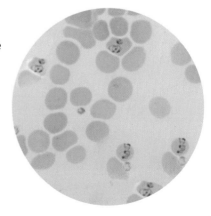

It was also known that there were a lot of mosquitoes in swampy areas, but no one made the connection. The period between a mosquito bite and the first symptoms appearing can be anywhere between 8 and 25 days, so there was no obvious link. Besides, in the era when miasma theory prevailed, there was no concept of "germs" or other tiny substances that could cause illness.

Breakthroughs were possible only after the invention of the microscope allowed scientists to see protozoa for the first time, when miasma theory began to fall out of favor in the 19th century. French military doctor Charles Louis Alphonse Laveran (1845–1922) noticed strange crescent-shape substances in the blood of malaria patients that were never present in those who did not have the disease, and that seemed to clear up after the administration of quinine, the active ingredient in cinchona bark. It was the first time a protozoan had been suggested as the cause of any disease, and Laveran's theories met a lot of resistance in the medical profession.

Laveran and his contemporaries believed that these protozoans were being inhaled from the air or ingested by drinking water. While working in India in the 1890s, a British army surgeon Ronald Ross found out that mosquitoes fed on blood infected with malaria took up the *Plasmodium* protozoa and passed them on, but most of his work was on birds. An Italian team was the first to confirm that *Anopheles* mosquitoes were the vector for transmission in humans—a revolutionary idea at the time.

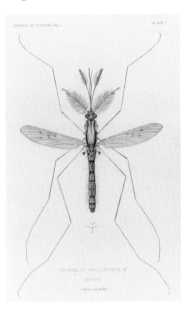

STILL A KILLER

Once the *Anopheles* mosquito had been identified as the vector for malaria, authorities could focus on controlling the mosquito population. The insecticide DDT was invented in 1874 and, during World War II, it was used to try to reduce the incidence of malaria among U.S. troops. Employed as an agricultural pesticide during the 1940s and 1950s, it helped to eliminate malaria from North America and Europe. However, in 1962 Rachel Carson wrote the highly influential book *Silent Spring*, in which she claimed that DDT can cause cancer and decimates wildlife, and amid growing concern it was banned in 1972. In the 21st century prevention remains the first resort, with antimalarial medicines as well as topical insecticides recommended for those visiting malarial regions.

Quinine was the standard treatment for malaria throughout the first half of the 20th century but it didn't stop 60,000 U.S. troops from dying

Anopheles atroparvus, thought to have been the main vector for spreading malaria through Europe in the early 20th century. The disease was eliminated from the United States in the 1950s and from the European Union in 1975; most reported cases there are now imported from tropical regions.

of the disease in Africa and the South Pacific during World War II. During the 1930s, a medicine called chloroquine was developed for both prevention and cure; it was first used after the war, but by the 1950s strains of malaria were developing that were resistant to it. At present, a cocktail of medicines is offered to those with malaria and foremost among them is artemisinin, derived from the artemisia plant that the Chinese used in antiquity. However, the overprescribing of malaria drugs in some countries is almost certain to produce more drug-resistant strains, so research continues, as does the hunt for a vaccine. According to the World Health Organization, there were 198 million cases in 2013, with between 584,000 and 855,000 deaths, of which 90 percent were in Africa.

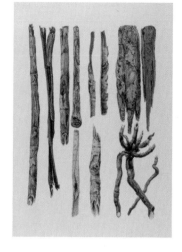

The powdered bark of Cinchona officinalis has many medicinal uses: as a muscle relaxant, a digestive stimulant, a fever reducer and a suppressor of heart palpitations.

> *It's going to be a very long war if for every division I have facing the enemy, I have one sick in hospital and another recovering from this dreadful disease.*
> —GENERAL DOUGLAS MACARTHUR, 1941

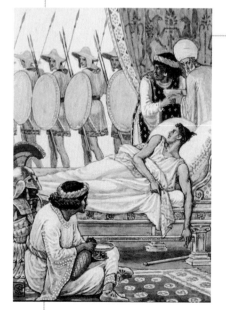

How Malaria Changed the World

Alexander the Great was killed by malaria at the age of 33, at the height of his powers. Had he lived and continued to rule over Greece, Arabia, the eastern Mediterranean and as far east as India, the world map might have looked completely different today. It is thought that Genghis Khan decided not to invade Western Europe because of the prevalence of malaria there at the time. Napoleon used malaria to attack British troops in 1809, when he flooded the Dutch countryside to allow the disease to become rampant. Of 240,000 deaths in the British ranks during that war, it is thought that only 30,000 died in battle, the rest from illness. During World War I, British, French and German troops in Macedonia were badly affected; when one French general was ordered to attack, he replied: "Regret that my army is in the hospital with malaria."

PROTOZOAN DISEASES

In the late 19th century, when building empires brought Western powers into Africa, India, and the Far East, more diseases caused by protozoa were encountered. Leishmaniasis, spread by protozoa in sand flies, is a particularly nasty one. The first symptom is raw skin lesions, followed by fever and ulcers both internally and externally. As with malaria, there are descriptions of the disease going back to antiquity, but it was in 1898 that Peter Borovsky in Tashkent first attributed the disease to protozoa. His research was not publicized, but in 1901 pathologist William Leishman found organisms in smears taken from the spleen of a patient who had died in India. Ronald Ross correctly identified them as protozoa and named them after Leishman. Leishmaniasis presented a huge problem for troops in Sicily during World War II. There is still no vaccine against it and the most effective drug treatments are expensive. Two million new cases are reported every year, with between 20,000 and 50,000 deaths.

Among the more puzzling diseases that white Europeans found in Africa was one that seemed to make people drowsy and confused, with difficulty walking and talking. While carrying out autopsies on patients who had died of this condition, Italian doctor Aldo Castellani discovered protozoa in their spinal fluid. The following year it was discovered that these protozoa, *Trypanosoma brucei*, were transmitted by the tsetse fly, and that their effect was to disrupt neurological pathways disrupting the sleep–wake cycle in those who succumb. In 2010 trypanosomiasis caused 9,000 deaths worldwide, most of them in the Democratic Republic of Congo.

Yellow Fever

Yellow fever gets its name because, left untreated, it causes liver damage, making the skin and the whites of the eyes yellow. There were devastating outbreaks in the United States and Central America throughout the 19th century. Cuban doctor Carlos Finlay realized in 1881 that it was mosquito borne. No one believed him until 1900 when American physician Walter Reed set up a controlled experiment to prove it. In 1904, one of his team, William C. Gorgas, was sent to help at the building of the Panama Canal, which was beleaguered by the number of workers succumbing to yellow fever and malaria. Gorgas drained all standing water, fumigated living quarters and provided mosquito netting for workers; and by 1906, the Canal Zone was free of yellow fever.

In March the pestilence spread with frightful rapidity and ... the greatest terror prevailed in all quarters of the town. The press endeavored to calm the fears of the inhabitants by publishing fewer deaths than took place ... nothing could exceed the gloom and desolation that pervaded the city.
—DR. J.H. SCRIVENER ON THE 1871 YELLOW FEVER OUTBREAK IN BUENOS AIRES, *MEDICAL TIMES AND GAZETTE*, 1872

Edward Jenner's Lancet

LOCATION: Berkeley, Gloucestershire, England
DATE: 1796
FIELD: Immunology

Smallpox was the leading cause of death in 18th-century Europe and was prevalent around the world. Those who survived an attack often suffered a range of permanent disabilities, from blindness and limb deformities to the characteristic pockmark scarring. It was every parent's worst nightmare that their child should catch it, and from monarchs to peasants all were desperate to find a cure. However, when the English country physician Edward Jenner suggested introducing the pus caused by a cow disease through tiny scratches cut with his lancet, he was mocked by scientists and pilloried in the press.

> *The smallpox was always present, filling the churchyards with corpses, tormenting with constant fears all whom it had stricken, leaving on those whose lives it spared the hideous traces of its power, turning the babe into a changeling at which the mother shuddered, and making the eyes and cheeks of the bighearted maiden objects of horror to the lover.*
>
> —THOMAS BABINGTON MACAULEY, *THE HISTORY OF ENGLAND FROM THE ACCESSION OF JAMES II, 1685–1702* (1848)

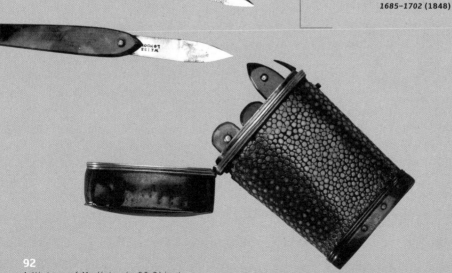

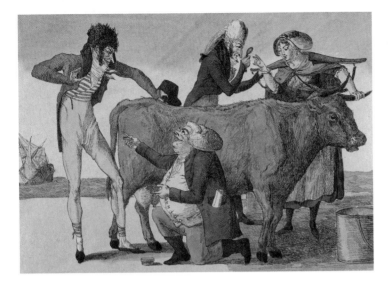

Edward Jenner's inoculation is mocked in a cartoon, ca. 1800: one physician inspects the cowpox lesions on a milkmaid's hand, while the gentleman farmer passes a lancet to a second physician.

FAMOUS VICTIMS

There is speculation that the smallpox virus originally crossed from rodents into the human population, and it is described in ancient Indian texts as early as 1500 BCE. Signs of the disease are detectable in the mummy of an Egyptian pharaoh, who died in 1145 BCE, and an epidemic in Japan in 735–737 CE is thought to have killed about one third of the population. Hippocrates did not mention smallpox, so it cannot have been common in Europe in his time, but there may have been an outbreak in Rome in 165–180 CE. It was certainly established across Europe by the 16th century, probably spread by the Crusaders, and when explorers crossed the Atlantic, they took it with them, devastating the native populations of the Americas.

Infection spread through droplets exhaled by people with the disease, or through contact with their bodily fluids on surfaces they had touched. Smallpox has an incubation period of 12 days, but those who catch it are not infectious until the fever and large flat pustules appear. Death comes within 10 to 16 days for those with a fatal dose of the ordinary virus, and within six days for those with hemorrhagic smallpox. No one was immune. It killed several monarchs, including Peter II of Russia,

Importing Disease

When the conquistadores crossed to the New World, they took with them a host of Old-World diseases to which the natives had no resistance, including smallpox, typhus, cholera and measles. Smallpox devastated the island of Hispaniola in 1507, before spreading to the Mexican mainland. When Hernán Cortés arrived in Tenochtitlán (modern-day Mexico City) in 1520, he found half the inhabitants had smallpox and the rest had either perished or fled. Disease moved faster than the invaders, so as the explorers advanced they found communities weakened by one or more of the dreaded European illnesses, making the Spanish conquest of the Aztecs and Incas much easier than it would otherwise have been. It's estimated that by 1595 more than 18 million had died, and some suggest that 95 percent of the native population of the Americas died of these new diseases during the 130 years after the invaders first arrived.

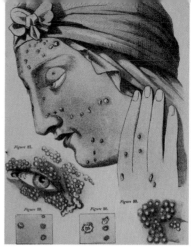

Louis XV of France, and Edward VI, the only son of Henry VIII of England. It killed the American Indian chief Sitting Bull, the Aztec chief Cuitláhuac and the Inca ruler Huayna Capac. George Washington, Mary Queen of Scots, and Joseph Stalin are among world leaders who survived the disease, although Stalin was notoriously self-conscious about the pockmarks he was left with.

FROM VARIOLATION TO VACCINATION

There are accounts as far back as the 10th century of the practice of variolation, whereby a small amount of pus extracted from a smallpox pustule was introduced through a scratch into the blood of someone as yet unaffected by the disease. It was hoped thus to stimulate them to develop resistance. The downsides were that they became infectious and could pass on smallpox to others, and some got ill themselves, with between 0.5 and 2 percent dying as a result of variolation. Many considered the risk worthwhile, because the disease itself had a mortality rate of 30 to 35 percent. Catherine the Great of Russia and her son were treated this way and both survived.

In English farming communities, there was an old wives' tale that those who became ill with cowpox never went on to catch smallpox. Edward Jenner, a Gloucestershire physician, made a study of dairy workers and became convinced that cowpox held the key to controlling smallpox. In 1796 he persuaded a farmer to let him inoculate his 8-year-old son, James Phipps, with cowpox, then 6 weeks later to introduce smallpox pus through two small cuts on his left arm. As he suspected, James Phipps had acquired immunity to smallpox.

Jenner did not understand how antibodies work and he could not identify the *Variola* virus that caused smallpox, because the microscopes of his day were not powerful enough to see them, but he knew his method was effective. He wrote to the Royal Society about his discovery but they told him he did not have enough proof. Jenner went on to inoculate

A smallpox rash began around the mouth and throat before spreading. Pustules in the eye could cause blindness, and in the respiratory system could cause pneumonia.

A cartoon of 1802 shows recipients of Edward Jenner's vaccine growing cows' heads on different parts of their anatomy. Despite the satirists, most were anxious to try the new vaccine in the hope of avoiding the epidemic that had killed about 400,000 Europeans in the late 18th century.

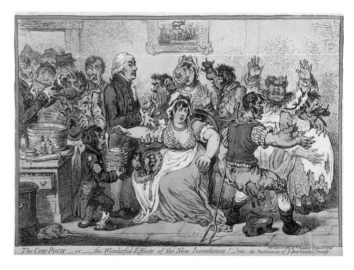

The Cow-Pock _ or _ the Wonderful Effects of the New Inoculation! _Vide. the Publications of ye Anti Vaccine Society_

23 others, including his own 11-month-old son, with the same results. He called the process vaccination, from the Latin word *vacca*, or "cow." The press ridiculed his methods, with many cartoonists showing people growing cows' heads after receiving Jenner's vaccination. However, by the end of 1801, 100,000 people across Great Britain had been vaccinated and incidence of the infection had started to fall dramatically.

ERADICATION

Word of Jenner's vaccine spread around the world and everyone wanted it. It was introduced to Newfoundland in 1800, to the Spanish colonies of South America in 1803, and in 1853 an Act of Parliament in the United Kingdom made smallpox vaccination compulsory. The numbers of cases began to drop steadily, but it did not die out as long as there were unvaccinated people to whom it could pass. By the mid-20th century, 10 million to 15 million people still caught the disease annually and two million of them died.

Concerted campaigns were begun to eradicate the disease completely. In 1950 there was a Pan American Health Organization campaign against smallpox, and in 1966 the World Health Organization (see pages 176–77) voted for a 10-year vaccination campaign. Using a process of "ring vaccination," they prevented outbreaks from spreading by isolating patients and vaccinating everyone who had been in contact with them.

Gradually, they achieved their goal. The last naturally occurring case of smallpox was in October 1975, when a 2-year-old Bangladeshi girl, Rahima Banu, contracted the disease and survived. In 1978 a laboratory worker Janet Parker accidentally caught it from a sample stored in the University of Birmingham medical school in England and died. Thereafter, all stocks worldwide were destroyed except for two: one in the United States Centers for Disease Control and Prevention in Atlanta, Georgia, and the other at a laboratory in Russia, where they remain to this day.

Anti-Vaccinationism

In the 1830s a vociferous minority began to protest about being told that they should have foreign substances introduced into their blood through vaccination. However, for a vaccine to stop the spread of an illness, between 85 and 95 percent of the population need to receive it. In 1905 the U.S. Supreme Court ruled that protecting the health of the nation through compulsory vaccination outweighed the individual's right to privacy. Throughout the 20th century, vaccines remained controversial among some alternative health practitioners, but effective new vaccines continued to be developed, including ones against measles, polio (see pages 160–63), and diphtheria. Today, the only major killer diseases for which no successful vaccines have yet been developed are HIV and malaria.

Future nations will know by history only that the loathsome small-pox has existed and by you has been extirpated.

—PRESIDENT THOMAS JEFFERSON, LETTER TO EDWARD JENNER, 1806

Laënnec's Stethoscope

LOCATION:	Paris, France
DATE:	1816
FIELD:	Cardiology, respiratory medicine, obstetrics

Auscultation, the practice of listening to sounds inside the body, was used as a diagnostic test back in ancient Greece and remained a basic technique for physicians in the early 19th century. That is when French physician René Laënnec had his brain wave and invented the stethoscope, which could amplify internal sounds and thus enable physicians to make more accurate diagnoses. His early stethoscope was a simple tube instead of the Y-shaped device we see strung around physicians' necks today, but it still got his name into the history books.

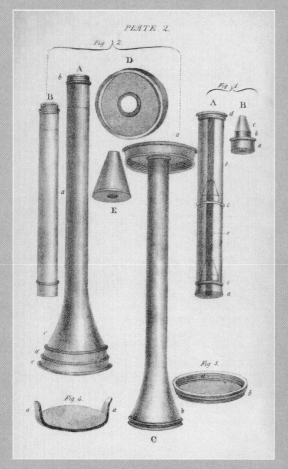

It must be confessed that there is something even ludicrous in the picture of a grave physician formally listening through a long tube applied to the patient's thorax, as if the disease within were a living being that could communicate its condition to the sense without.

—DR. JOHN FORBES, ENGLISH TRANSLATOR OF LAËNNEC'S *TREATISE ON DISEASES OF THE CHEST*, 1821

THE LISTENING EAR

The story goes that one day Laënnec was presented with a particularly plump female patient with a heart condition. It seemed wrong to place his head on her ample chest, so he rolled up a sheaf of papers in imitation of the ear trumpets then in use. Listening to her heart through the tube, he realized sounds could be heard "with much greater clearness and distinctness that I had ever done before." Laënnec designed a wooden tube, 12 inches (30 cm) long and ¾ inch (2 cm) in diameter, in three parts, which he called a "stethoscope," from the Greek words *stethos* ("chest") and *skopein* ("to see").

With his new listening device, Laënnec went on to describe the chest sounds he heard and to link them to specific diseases. This had personal significance for him, because tuberculosis (see pages 102–105) had killed his mother; it would, in fact, lead to his own death at the age of 45.

Wooden stethoscopes were replaced with ones made of pliable tubing, and in 1852 American physician George P. Cammann added two earpieces and a bell-shape end to place on the chest, giving binaural sound. In 1878 a microphone was connected to stethoscopes, and in 1895 Adolphe Pinard invented a stethoscope that could listen to fetal heartbeats. By the 1970s, electronic stethoscopes could even produce graphs of the heartbeat.

Following the introduction of x-rays and other types of scans (see pages 194–97), the stethoscope was less relied upon but it is still used in most physicians' offices as a first-line method of detecting problems with the heart and lungs.

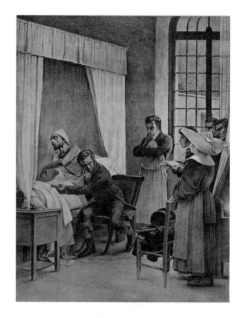

René Laënnec using his stethoscope on a patient in the Necker hospital in Paris, France, in 1816.

Diagnosing Sounds

Laënnec described several different chest sounds, including:

- **Rales, a clicking, rattling sound on inhalation as air gets into spaces normally closed to airflow; heard in patients with pneumonia or congestive heart failure**
- **Wheezing, the high-pitched whistle on exhalation that indicates obstructed bronchial tubes, as in asthma, bronchitis or chronic obstructive pulmonary disease**
- **Stridor, the harsh vibratory sound of an obstructed trachea, which could indicate croup or a foreign body trapped there.**

A normal heart has a regular sound described as "lub-dub," but Laënnec showed that a slight whooshing can indicate a heart murmur caused by irregularity in the blood flow through the heart.

Morton's Ether Inhaler

LOCATION: Boston, Massachusetts
DATE: 1846
FIELD: Surgery, pharmacology, physiology

Oh, what delight for every feeling heart to find the new year ushered in with the announcement of this noble discovery of the power to still the sense of pain, and veil the eye and memory from all the horrors of an operation. We have conquered pain!

—REPORT ON THE USE OF ETHER, **PEOPLE'S JOURNAL, 1847**

The use of anesthetics to allow painless and safer surgery did not hail from a single "Eureka!" moment but instead from the work of dozens of men over the centuries and across continents. In 1846 Boston dentist William Morton declared himself the first to demonstrate publicly the use of ether as a surgical anesthetic and even tried to patent ether under the name "Letheon." However, many others could lay claim to being "fathers of anesthesia," back to the Sumerians of ancient Mesopotamia.

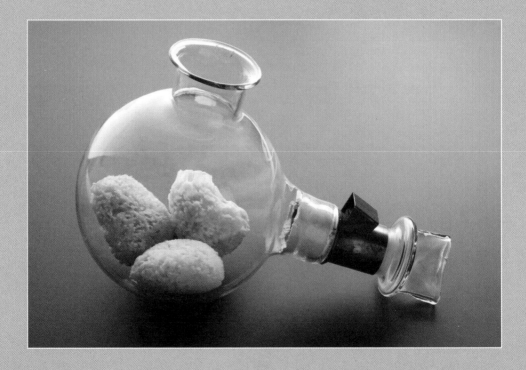

HENBANE AND MANDRAKE ROOT

Anesthetics used in the ancient world included alcohol, opium, henbane and mandrake root, but all of these had drawbacks—not least that an overdose could be fatal. Alcohol and possibly opium are said to have been used in Sumer ca. 3400 BCE. About 300 BCE Chinese surgeon Bian Que gave two men a drink that made them sleep for 3 days, during which time he performed gastric surgery on them, but the ingredients of his potion have not survived. Avicenna's *Canon of Medicine*, written ca. 1020 CE, describes a "soporific sponge" containing narcotics and aromatics that was placed under a patient's nose during surgery to promote sleep. However, throughout the Renaissance, operations remained a last resort and few were even attempted: amputations, removal of bladder stones and visible cancerous tumors, and surface procedures were performed, but the chest, head and abdomen would be opened only in situations of life or death.

Eastern and Western medicine took different approaches to the problem of how to control pain during surgery. In 1804 Hanaoka Seishu of Osaka, Japan, anesthetized a 60-year-old woman using a herbal formula he called *tsusensan* and was able to perform a successful mastectomy on her. Among his ingredients were parts of the angelica plant, containing active chemicals that would certainly have had an anesthetic effect. He performed more than 30 operations using *tsusensan*. In the West the approach switched from ingestion of soporific substances to inhalation after Humphry Davy discovered the anesthetic qualities of a gas first isolated by Joseph Priestley in 1774: nitrous oxide.

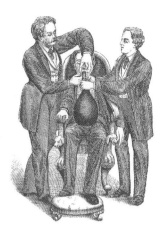

Samuel Lee Rymer, a dentist in the London suburb of Croydon, administers nitrous oxide to a patient in 1863. Rymer was instrumental in the founding of a Society of Dentists and a College of Dentistry in England.

Opium

Extract of the white poppy *Papaver somniferum* was used for pain relief in antiquity and is mentioned by many early medical writers, including Avicenna and Galen. During the mid-17th century, British herbalist Thomas Sydenham dissolved opium in alcohol to make the highly addictive laudanum that inspired the Romantic poets Coleridge and Shelley. In 1805 Friedrich Sertürner isolated morphine from opium and named it after Morpheus, the Roman god of dreams. Decades later, pharmaceutical company Bayer produced heroin in 1898 and advertised it as "the heroic drug." Trade wars broke out with China as Europeans and Americans clamored to secure ample supplies of the precious poppy. By 1900, it is estimated that 250,000 Americans were addicted to its calming, narcotic effects.

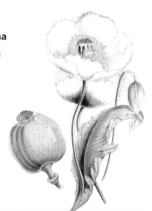

ETHER PARTIES

After Humphry Davy demonstrated in 1799 that inhaling nitrous oxide made people relaxed and giggly, "laughing gas" was used to entertain guests at fashionable parties on both sides of the Atlantic. In 1815 Michael Faraday showed that ether had the same effects, and ether parties were all the rage. By mid-century, chloroform became another party drug, with no one seeming to appreciate that these substances could be lethal in overdose.

Several practitioners claimed to have been the first to use anesthetic gas during surgery. In 1824 Henry Hickman published the results of his trials of carbon dioxide and nitrous oxide used to anesthetize animals for surgery. In 1842 Crawford Long of Georgia administered ether to a boy called James Venable before excising a growth from his neck, but he did not publish a report of his work until 1849, by which time William Morton had already claimed his place in the history books.

In 1846, at Massachusetts General Hospital, Morton anesthetized a man who was having a tumor removed from his jaw, using ether administered through an inhaler. After the operation, he changed the color and smell of the gas he had used and attempted to market it as Letheon, but doctors were not fooled. Morton spent the rest of his life attempting to defend his position as the "inventor" of anesthesia.

Top-Speed Amputations

Before the invention of antibiotics, limb amputations were the only answer doctors had to the sepsis that invariably resulted from mud-encrusted battlefield wounds, but before the days of effective anesthesia the procedure was brutal and more often than not fatal. The mortality rate in 1842 was 62 percent for amputations through the thigh, with death occurring as a result of hemorrhage, sepsis, or shock. The patient would be pinned down and given a slug of alcohol before the surgeon began. A tourniquet would be applied before the limb was hewn off, and the veins and arteries were tied with ligatures. Speed was of the essence and in 1846, Scottish surgeon Robert Liston boasted that he could complete a leg amputation in an average of 2½ minutes.

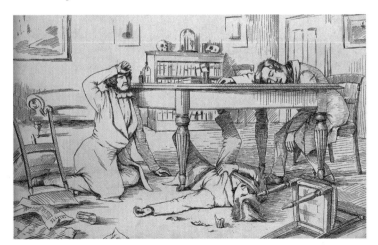

Scottish obstetrician James Young Simpson and his friends, Dr. Keith and Dr. Duncan, experiment with liquid chloroform, 1840s. They experienced euphoria at first before falling asleep until morning, whereupon Simpson realized it would be useful as an anesthetic.

ETHER, CHLOROFORM, AND COCAINE

Ether had several disadvantages as an anesthetic. It made people cough and feel nauseated when they inhaled it, and it was also highly flammable, which was not ideal in the days when homes and doctors' offices were lit by candles and gas lamps. Chloroform seemed an improvement at first. It was dripped as a liquid onto a cloth held over the patient's face or administered via an inhaler, but it was found to slow the heartbeat and could cause heart failure and liver damage. One in 2,500 patients died from chloroform anesthetics, whereas just one in 15,000 died from ether. Both left the patient feeling nauseous and groggy when they came around, and were not universally popular at first.

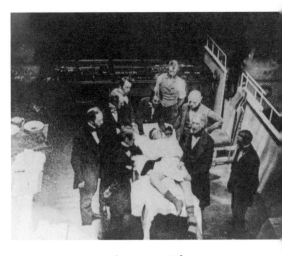

A reenactment of the demonstration of anesthesia with ether inhalation by William Morton on October 16, 1846, watched by a group of surgeons. The patient, Mr. Edward Gilbert Abbott, experienced no pain as a tumor was removed from his jaw.

British anesthetist and epidemiologist John Snow (see pages 106–109) believed in using the lowest dosage possible, and when he was selected to attend Queen Victoria during the birth of her eighth and ninth children, he used just a couple of drops of chloroform. Once news got around that the great queen had endorsed anesthesia, its popularity began to increase.

Cocaine was first isolated from coca leaves in 1859, and New York physician William Halsted realized that, when injected into the nerves, it could anesthetize local areas. He experimented on himself, and ended up addicted to cocaine—but by then he had invented the principle of local anesthetic. German researcher August Bier injected cocaine solution into the spinal fluid of his colleague August Hildebrandt to anesthetize the lower body, and he demonstrated the absence of pain by hammering his partner's shins and burning him with a lit cigar.

Modern anesthetics use a combination of drugs to relax the muscles, relieve pain and promote unconsciousness. Tracheal intubation (inserting a tube into the windpipe) allows accurate control of dosage, and monitors check the breathing and heart rate of patients while they are sedated. This allows for longer, more painstaking operations. The world's longest took place over 4 days in 1951 when surgeons removed a 150-pound (68-kg) ovarian cyst from a Michigan woman. The death rate from general anesthesia is now less than one in 250,000.

> *All pain is per se and especially in excess, destructive and ultimately fatal in its nature and effects.*
>
> **—JAMES YOUNG SIMPSON, 1847**

TB Sanatorium in Görbersdorf

LOCATION: Görbersdorf, Germany (now Sokołowsko, Poland)
DATE: 1854
FIELD: Respiratory diseases, bacteriology, epidemiology

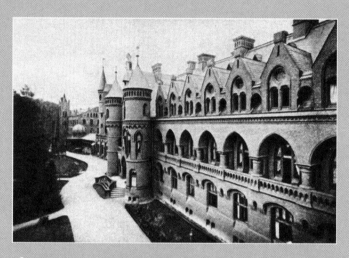

A ghostly complexion, fever, a recurrent cough, blood-tinged sputum and weight loss were symptoms of one of the most dreaded diseases of the 18th and 19th centuries, which killed one in four people across Europe. Its ancient Greek name was phthisis, but it was commonly called consumption, and to physicians it was tuberculosis (TB). Some thought it was caused by vampires, others by emotional stress, yet more believed it hereditary, and many blamed the poor for not keeping their homes clean enough—but no one had a cure. Then in the mid-19th century the imposing figure of Hermann Brehmer opened the first TB sanatorium; the strict routine he recommended would be popular among TB patients for the next hundred years.

> *This disease isn't dangerous at my age, and they say the cure is going on quite well, though slowly ... We are now sending for some new American drug called streptomycin which they say will speed up the cure.*
>
> —ENGLISH NOVELIST GEORGE ORWELL, WRITING FROM HAIRMYRES HOSPITAL, SCOTLAND, 1948

THE KING'S EVIL

Mycobacterium tuberculosis, which causes TB, has been found in Neolithic skeletons and Egyptian mummies. Hippocrates called it the most widespread disease of his day and said it was invariably fatal. Traditional bloodletting treatments weakened already frail invalids and hastened their end, but no one knew what else to try.

In medieval times they called scrofula—a swelling of the lymph glands associated with tuberculosis—"the king's evil" and thought it could be cured by the touch of a monarch. In the 11th century, Edward the Confessor of England and Philip I of France became the first monarchs to touch scrofula patients, and many more followed. Despite growing evidence that the disease was contagious, the practice continued until 1825 in France, although the weight of evidence must have made it clear by then that those who had been touched by kings were not surviving any longer than those who had not.

During the 19th century, as industrialization took hold in the Western world, country folk flocked to the expanding cities and tuberculosis spread rapidly in the cramped, insanitary conditions of slums. In one in 10 cases, the TB bacteria lie latent in the body and the patient remains symptomless but still infectious, which makes the disease particularly insidious. Infection is spread by respiratory fluids in the air or left on surfaces, and if the disease becomes active, it kills 50 percent of patients who do not receive treatment.

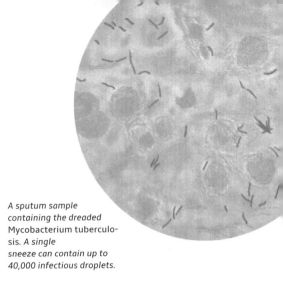

A sputum sample containing the dreaded Mycobacterium tuberculosis. *A single sneeze can contain up to 40,000 infectious droplets.*

The White Plague

During the 19th century, tuberculosis acquired a romantic reputation as a number of famous musicians, artists, and writers succumbed: John Keats, Emily and Anne Brontë, and Chopin, among others. It was a long, drawn-out death that gave patients ample time to consider their own mortality and prepare for the afterlife, in a way that concentrated the mind. "I should like to die of consumption," Lord Byron wrote, and society ladies whitened their faces to create a consumptive appearance.

Twentieth-century victims included Franz Kafka, who received treatment in a Viennese sanatorium, and George Orwell, who died in 1950 after being unable to tolerate the side effects of streptomycin.

In February 1820 poet John Keats coughed up a little blood and declared "It is arterial blood ... my death warrant." The treatment prescribed was near starvation and frequent bloodletting. He died in February 1821.

THE SANATORIUM EXPERIENCE

While at medical school, Hermann Brehmer wrote in a thesis on tuberculosis that he believed people with the disease had small hearts relative to the size of their lungs, and the lungs were therefore not receiving an adequate blood supply. He proposed that the lower levels of oxygen found in air at high altitude would enlarge the heart and improve the health of patients. Brehmer had contracted TB himself and found his condition vastly improved by a visit to the Himalayas. He settled in Görbersdorf, a German town at an altitude of 2,000 feet (600 m), and in 1862 he opened his *Heilenstalt* (German for "healing place"), with 40 beds for TB patients.

However much the sanatorium resembled other institutions, it had one unique feature—the omnipresence of the shadow of death .... Staff tried to brush it off with aphorisms about being strong and determined. But in countless ways, some personal, others collective, the sanatorium experience was at its core an encounter with mortality.

—SHEILA ROTHMAN, *LIVING IN THE SHADOW OF DEATH*, 1994

The routine at Görbersdorf was strict, with supervised exercise, mountain walks, wet rubdowns and cold showers. Brehmer served patients wine with their dinner and cognac at bedtime, which he thought would strengthen their hearts, and he made them record their temperatures every 2 hours. During the first decade after it opened, Görbersdorf took 958 patients, and the mortality rate was an incredibly low 4.8 percent. Brehmer's treatments did not in themselves constitute a cure but they stimulated the immune systems of his patients, helping them to fight the disease. Görbersdorf's reputation grew, and by 1904 it was the largest sanatorium in the world, with 300 beds.

A ward at Stannington Sanitorium in Northumberland, the first British sanatorium for children with tuberculosis. It opened in 1908 and could accommodate 11,000 patients.

One of Brehmer's patients, Peter Dettweiler, opened his own sanatorium in Falkenstein in 1876, and the only change from Brehmer's routine was that he advocated plenty of bed rest. During the 1870s, the first U.S. sanatorium was opened in the Appalachian Mountains by Joseph Gleitsmann, and by 1953 there were 839 facilities across the United States advocating fresh air, sunshine, plenty of bed rest and a healthy diet.

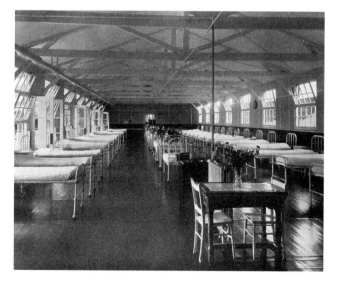

TOWARD A CURE

The key to understanding what caused TB began with René Laënnec's work on identifying the disease through auscultation of the chest (see pages 96–97) and his demonstration that the pulmonary lesions found in autopsy caused the symptoms experienced by living patients. In 1865 Jean-Antoine Villemin proved that the disease was transmissible, and in 1882 Robert Koch (see pages 117–18) identified the tuberculosis bacillus but failed to find an effective test or cure for TB. The development of x-rays by Wilhelm Röntgen (see pages 132–37) allowed doctors to track the progress of the disease in patients, and in 1907 Clemens von Pirquet developed a skin test for it—but still there was no cure.

During the early years of the 20th century, surgical treatments were tried that involved collapsing parts of the lungs to rest the infected areas and allow lesions to heal. Some of these operations were brutal, involving the removal of ribs, which left the patients hunchbacked and with uneven shoulders; these procedures were not particularly effective.

A vaccine developed by Albert Calmette and Camille Guérin from the bovine strain of tuberculosis was first tried on humans in 1921. Known as the BCG (Bacillus Calmette–Guérin), it greatly reduced the incidence of the disease once its use became widespread after World War II. In 1944 an antibiotic (see pages 164–67) called streptomycin was developed; this proved successful against *M. tuberculosis*, and it was followed by isoniazid in 1952. The number of cases plummeted until the 1980s when a drug-resistant strain of tuberculosis emerged and the spread of HIV (see pages 202–205) triggered a resurgence among those with weakened immune systems. In the 21st century, TB remains the world's second most deadly infectious disease, after HIV.

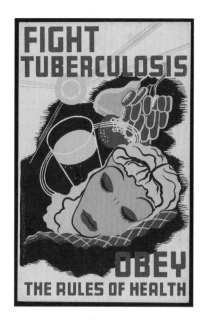

A 1936 poster advising sun exposure, a healthy diet and plenty of sleep to prevent tuberculosis. The public were also warned to avoid spitting in public places, which could spread the bacteria.

Routine at Catawba Sanatorium, Roanoke, Virginia, 1920

7:15	**Rising bell**
8:00 to 8:30	**Breakfast**
8:30 to 11:00	**Rest or exercise as ordered**
11:00 to 12:45	**Rest on bed**
1:00 to 1:30	**Dinner**
1:45 to 4:00	**Rest on bed, reading but no talking allowed. Quiet hour.**
4:00 to 5:45	**Rest or exercise as ordered**
6:00	**Supper**
8:00	**Nourishment if ordered**
9:00	**All patients in pavilions**
9:30	**All lights out**

John Snow's Cholera Map

LOCATION:	London, England
DATE:	1854
FIELD:	Epidemiology

The lips blue, the face haggard, the eyes hollow, the stomach sunk in, the limbs contracted and crumpled as if by fire, those are the signs of the great illness which, invoked by a malediction of the priests, comes down to slay the brave.

—TEMPLE INSCRIPTION IN GUJARAT, INDIA, 400–300 BCE

A cholera-like disease was reported in India back in ancient times, but it was during the 19th century, when trade routes opened up between Europe, Russia and the Americas, that it began to spread around the world. The symptoms were horrific, with severe diarrhea soon leading to dehydration. The severity of the onset was terrifying and around half of all people with cholera perished within days—or in some cases hours. Most scientists believed that disease was caused by "miasma" or foul vapors in the air, but a London-based obstetrician called John Snow decided to dig a little deeper.

CHOLERA PANDEMICS

In 1817 heavy rainfall led to severe flooding across India, and with it came a particularly devastating cholera outbreak. It quickly spread around the countries of southeast Asia and as far as the Arabian peninsula before dying down in 1823, but not before hundreds of thousands had perished in acute agony. The first symptoms they experienced were faintness and sweating, followed by acute cramps and watery diarrhea. Within hours, victims could become so severely dehydrated that they died an agonizing death.

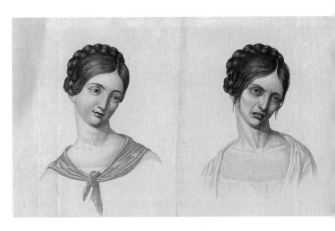

A young woman depicted before and after contracting cholera. Her skin and lips have turned blue from lack of oxygen and her sunken cheeks indicate dehydration.

During a second pandemic in 1829–33, the disease reached China, Russia, Europe and North America. It was probably carried across the Atlantic by Irish emigrants, and by 1833 it had reached Latin America. The third pandemic, which would be the deadliest of all, began in India in 1852 and over the next 7 years it spread virtually worldwide, killing over a million people. In England alone, 23,000 people died in 1854.

Governments tried imposing quarantine measures, as had been done during the plague, but this did not seem to make a difference. Treatment by bloodletting did nothing. Calomel, or mercury chloride, was prescribed as a purgative to rid the body of the disease but it must have increased the agony. The only other treatment tried was opium, which would have reduced the pain of the cramps but done nothing to effect a cure. Doctors were stumped.

JOHN SNOW'S DETECTIVE WORK

It was clear that the poor were more at risk of catching cholera than the rich, leading to claims that it was caused by exposure to filth and decay in their insanitary living conditions. Mysteriously, it didn't seem to be contagious in the way that previous plagues had been, because doctors could treat patients without falling ill themselves.

Cause of Death

After an incubation period that could be as little as 2 hours or as much as 5 days, those who caught cholera would be struck down without warning as the cramps and diarrhea began. They would feel desperately thirsty but drinking brought on violent vomiting; they would soon lose as much as one quarter of their body weight through dehydration, causing sunken eyes. The blood thickened and skin turned blue from lack of oxygenation, while the loss of electrolytes, especially potassium, caused the electrical impulses in the heart to falter, leading to death. In some cases, a person could appear healthy one moment and die just a few hours later.

London obstetrician and pioneer of anesthesia (see page 101), John Snow was fascinated by the disease, and after an 1848 outbreak in England he wrote a pamphlet about it. He observed that since it attacked the digestive system first, that pointed to the cause being ingested, whereas if it had been caused by miasma in the air one would expect the lungs to be affected first. Snow surmised that the families of cholera patients might be catching it when they accidentally ingested particles of diarrhea or vomit that had been left on sheets or clothing, and he also posited accurately that outbreaks were caused by water that had become contaminated by feces.

In July 1854 there was a renewed cholera outbreak in London. Between August 29 and September 11, nearly 700 people died in a small, overcrowded area of Soho, where there were houses, workshops and taverns. Snow created a geographical grid indicating each cholera death and found they were clustered in an area just 500 yards (450 m) across, centered around the Broad Street water pump. He told local officials of his theory and with difficulty persuaded them to remove the handle of the pump. Three days later the epidemic ended.

THE BROAD STREET SURVEY

A Board of Health inquiry into the 1854 outbreak ignored the evidence that the pump was implicated and blamed "some atmospheric or widely diffused agent still to be discovered." However, the local church of St. Luke decided to hold its own inquiry, with John Snow's help, and set out to interview residents to find out why some had been infected and others had not. They discovered that of 137 people who had drunk from the Broad Street water pump, 80 had caught cholera. Of 297 others who lived nearby but had not drunk from the pump, only 20 caught cholera. This latter group included workers at the Broad Street brewery who drank from the brewery's own well—or drank the beer it made. The findings seemed fairly conclusive.

One case puzzled John Snow: An aunt and niece who lived some distance from Soho had died of cholera. When he talked to the woman's

> *Want of cleanliness was by no means more characteristic of the diseased than of the survivors.*
>
> **—REVEREND HENRY WHITEHEAD (WHO ASSISTED SNOW IN TRACING THE SOURCE OF THE OUTBREAK), 1855**

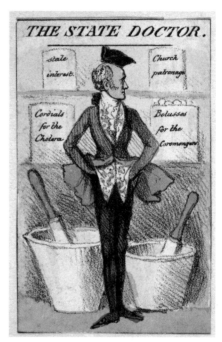

In this cartoon, the state is compared to a doctor peddling ineffective remedies for the country's ills, such as a cordial for cholera. Many such cordials, containing fruits, spices, herbs and salts, were marketed in the 19th century. They were not a cure but may have helped to rehydrate and restore electrolyte balance if the patient could keep them down.

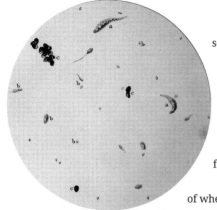

son, he was told that she used to live in Broad Street and liked the taste of the water from that pump so much that she had bottles of it delivered to her. One bottle had been filled on August 31; they both drank from it and died the following day.

There still remained the question of where the initial outbreak originated. Reverend Henry Whitehead, one of the investigators, discovered that the first victim of the Soho outbreak had been a 5-month-old baby girl who lived next to the pump. Her mother had washed her dirty diapers and dumped the water in a privy, which leaked into the well feeding the water pump, and the infection spread from there. Snow, who had long suspected poor sewage disposal, was vindicated.

Vibrio cholerae, the comma-shape bacilli, observed under the microscope. Humans can become infected by drinking water contaminated with feces, eating contaminated fish or shellfish, or not reheating leftover grains, such as rice, sufficiently before consumption.

IDENTIFYING THE CHOLERA BACILLUS

When he looked closely at the water from the Broad Street pump, Snow could see white flecks in it, and he suspected those might be the cause of the disease. He was not able to identify them; that honor went to Robert Koch in 1884 (see pages 117–18). He found that the cholera bacillus multiplied in warm, moist conditions, and that it was never found in the intestines of patients who died of other diarrhea-causing diseases.

For a long time the scientific community remained reluctant to abandon the miasma theory. At an international conference in 1874, scientists voted unanimously that "ambient air is the principal vehicle of the generative agent of cholera." However, the tide of opinion began to turn in the following decades thanks to the fastidious work of John Snow and the St. Luke's Church team. Their findings were influential in public health initiatives to build a safe system of sewage disposal and Snow's methods still form the basis for many epidemiological studies today.

Posthumous Fame

Italian scientist Filippo Pacini first discovered the cholera bacillus while examining under a microscope the intestinal mucus of patients who had died of the disease. He called the comma-shaped organisms he could see *Vibrio* and published a paper about them in 1854, but it was ignored by the scientific community and John Snow does not appear to have heard of it. Pacini also identified the cause of death as massive loss of fluid and electrolytes and recommended that patients be treated with an intravenous injection of salt water—a strategy that later proved to be most effective. In 1965 the name *Vibrio cholerae* was adopted to honor Pacini's early work.

Florence Nightingale's Lamp

LOCATION:	Scutari (now part of Istanbul, Turkey)
DATE:	1854–55
FIELD:	Nursing

Women were excluded from practicing as physicians in the 14th century, when it was ruled that a medical degree from a university was required and universities opted not to admit them. Guilds, such as the Barber-Surgeons, would not take women members either, so the only option for those drawn to the caring profession was to look after loved ones and neighbors. By the beginning of the 19th century, lower-class women were employed to clean and feed patients in public hospitals, but it would have been considered scandalous for a woman of any social position to attend a strange man lying in bed. Then along came Florence Nightingale, the "lady with the lamp," to blow away engrained attitudes and establish the modern profession of nursing.

I attribute my success to this—I never gave nor took any excuse.
—FLORENCE NIGHTINGALE

FROM PRAYING TO NURSING

Religious orders had long taken in the sick, with nuns working in convent infirmaries from medieval times. The Hôtel-Dieu in Paris (see pages 40–43) was run by Augustinian sisters, and women helped out in menial roles at many early hospitals. By the 19th century, however, the largely untrained women working in London's teeming hospitals had a bad reputation; Charles Dickens caricatured them as drunken, promiscuous and uncaring. Many female mid-wives had been forced out of business by men (see pages 76–81) and the folk wisdom of local "wise women" was usually dismissed in doctors' manuals as "old wives' tales."

The early 19th century saw a new generation of women who yearned to break free of the restraints of polite society and help the sick. In 1836 the Reverend Theodor Fliedner set up an influential 3-year course in Kaiserswerth (now part of Düsseldorf), Germany, where nurses could be trained in patient care. British social reformer Elizabeth Fry visited Kaiserswerth and it inspired her to establish an Institute of Nursing to train women of the Anglican faith in London. In 1851 Florence Nightingale also went to Kaiserswerth and on her return she took a job as superintendent of a hospital for sick gentlewomen in London's Harley Street—but her finest hour was yet to come.

When news flowed back from the Crimean War that British soldiers were dying in the thousands, mostly from disease instead of their battle wounds, and that both the French and Russian armies had "Sisters of Charity" to nurse them whereas the British did not, Florence Nightingale was incensed. In November 1854 she took a band of women out to Scutari (now part of Istanbul, Turkey) to set up her Barrack Hospital, and in the process became a British national heroine.

Mary Seacole

Jamaican-born Mary Seacole had nursed British soldiers in Panama and Cuba during the 1830s and 1840s, curing them of cholera and yellow fever with her mixture of herbal remedies and careful nursing. When there was a cholera outbreak in the first months of the Crimean War, she offered to travel there to help, but the British government refused because of the color of her skin. Undeterred, Mary Seacole sailed there under her own steam and set up her "British Hotel," where home cooking and herbal cures were dispensed to those in need. Her habit of venturing out onto the field of battle to treat the wounded made her extremely popular with the soldiers.

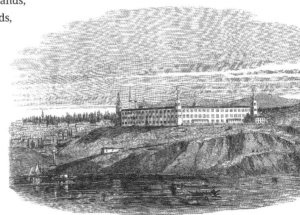

The Barrack Hospital in Scutari, part of modern-day Istanbul, where Florence Nightingale and her team of nurses treated soldiers wounded during the Crimean War of 1854–56.

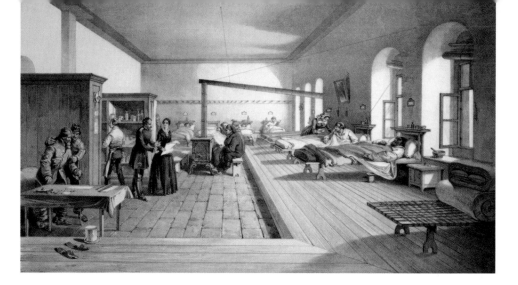

WARTIME NURSING

Florence Nightingale did not understand that microscopic "germs" might be responsible for disease, but all the same she was a great believer in cleanliness and on arrival she had the Barrack Hospital scrubbed from top to bottom. Windows were opened wide to let in air, and nutritious meals were served. What she did not know was that the hospital was built over an old sewer that contained decomposing animals, and at first the survival rate in her hospital was poor, but once the drains were cleared it improved dramatically. She banned her nurses from the wards at night for the sake of propriety but toured them herself, holding a Turkish fanoos lantern and dispensing comfort to the wounded. On her return to England, she opened a school of nursing at St. Thomas' Hospital in London and wrote an influential book entitled *Notes on Nursing* (1859), which set out a curriculum for nurses in training.

During the American Civil War of 1861–65, 3,000 women, most of them with no experience outside the home, nursed soldiers who were wounded. The mental health campaigner Dorothea Dix was appointed superintendent of Union Army nurses, and her decision that injured Confederate soldiers brought to her hospitals should receive care that was just as good as that given to their own side brought her universal respect. Antislavery campaigner Harriet Tubman ran a Civil War hospital on an island off South Carolina, and Clara Barton (see page 126) worked in a number of

A ward at the Barrack Hospital: Florence Nightingale learned a lot about sanitation from her work there, but still 80 percent of the British soldiers who died in the war perished of disease instead of their injuries.

> *Medicine is so broad a field, so closely interwoven with general interests, dealing as it does with all ages, sexes and classes, and yet of so personal a character in its individual appreciations, that it must be regarded as one of those great departments of work in which the cooperation of men and women is needed to fulfill all its requirements.*
>
> —ELIZABETH BLACKWELL, *PIONEER WORK IN OPENING THE MEDICAL PROFESSION TO WOMEN*, 1895

hospitals just behind the front lines of the great battles. These women's names became legendary and helped change attitudes toward women working in medicine. There was still a long way to go, but America's first school of nursing was established in Philadelphia in 1872.

WOMEN DOCTORS

One Crimean War hospital had a survival rate that was consistently higher than Florence Nightingale's. It was run by Dr. James Barry, who had trained in medicine at Edinburgh University in Scotland, served with distinction at the Battle of Waterloo (1815) and become Inspector-General of British military hospitals. It was only after dying of dysentery in 1865 that Dr. Barry was discovered to be a woman, Margaret Bulkley, making her the UK's first qualified female doctor.

British-born Elizabeth Blackwell was able to study at the Geneva Medical College in New York only because, when students were given a vote on whether she could attend, they thought it was a joke and voted yes. She graduated top of her class in 1849 but couldn't find work in a hospital, so she and her sister started their own, the New York Infirmary for Indigent Women and Children. She later moved to London, where she established a School of Medicine for Women in 1874 and worked with Elizabeth Garrett Anderson, the first British woman to qualify as a doctor in her own right. Unable to enter the profession by a direct route, Garrett Anderson had gained a license from the Society of Apothecaries, then went to Paris to take her final medical examination. It was as a result of her campaigning that women were finally allowed to study medicine at British universities from 1876. The tide turned across the world to the extent that in many countries there are now more female medical students than male.

Pioneering Women Doctors

Dorothea Erxleben gained a medical degree from the University of Halle, Germany, in 1754 after getting a special dispensation to study from Emperor Frederick the Great. In Sweden, Lovisa Åhrberg was successfully treating patients throughout the 1840s; when she was arrested and charged with being a "quack," her medical knowledge so impressed those sent to examine her that she was given an honorary licence to practice and a medal from the king. Rebecca Lee Crumpler was the first African American woman to qualify as a doctor after graduating in Boston, Massachusetts, in 1864, a time when it was still rare for black men to be admitted to medical schools, let alone women.

Three pioneering women in medicine: Elizabeth Blackwell, the first woman to qualify as a doctor in the United States, Elizabeth Garrett Anderson, who was the first female qualified doctor in England; and Scottish doctor Sophia Jex-Blake, who led the campaign for women to be allowed university educations.

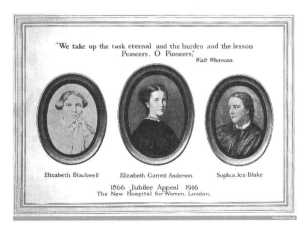

"We take up the task eternal and the burden and the lesson Pioneers. O Pioneers."

Walt Whitman.

Elizabeth Blackwell   Elizabeth Garrett Anderson   Sophia Jex-Blake

1866 Jubilee Appeal 1916
The New Hospital for Women, London.

Louis Pasteur's Flask

LOCATION:	France
DATE:	1859
FIELD:	Microbiology

The mid-19th century saw major leaps forward in several different fields of medicine, but perhaps the most significant was the gradual acceptance of the theory that many diseases were caused by living microorganisms, not Galen's miasma. Improvements in microscope technology meant that microbes could be seen, but which ones caused disease? The climate was competitive and researchers raced to publish their work before rivals could preempt them. One of the giants of the age was French microbiologist and chemist Louis Pasteur. Although best known today for inventing pasteurization, he made many original discoveries, some using his ingenious swan-neck flask. He may have occasionally taken shortcuts in his laboratory work and passed off others' research as his own, however, this does not remotely lessen his historical importance.

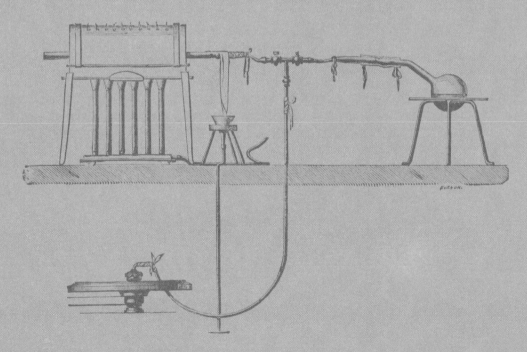

GERM THEORY

In the first century BCE, Roman scholar Marcus Terentius Varro had postulated that malaria (see pages 86–91) might be caused by "minute creatures which cannot be seen by the eyes," but he was centuries ahead of his time and his theory was largely ignored by contemporaries. In 1546 Italian physician Girolamo Fracastoro wrote an essay in which he proposed that inanimate substances such as clothes could foster the "essential seeds of contagion" and thus cause infection, but he also received scant attention. When some of Van Leeuwenhoek's "animalcules" (see page 82) were spotted in the blood of the sick when viewed under a microscope, it was at first assumed that they were a symptom. It was a huge leap from that premise to proving that these microorganisms actually caused disease.

Gradually the tide began to turn. In 1835 Italian entomologist Agostino Bassi discovered that a silkworm disease known as muscardine was caused by tiny living spores. Hungarian physician Ignaz Semmelweis established in the 1840s that contamination on the hands of medical students was causing puerperal fever (see page 81). In 1854 John Snow postulated that white substances in infected water were the cause of cholera (see page 109). But the two key figures who established the proof of what came to be known as "germ theory" were Louis Pasteur and his rival, German physician Robert Koch.

The Swan-neck Flask

The theory of spontaneous generation (see page 84) still prevailed in Pasteur's day, but he did not believe it. When the French Academy of Sciences offered a prize of 2,500 francs to anyone who could settle the matter, Pasteur devised a neat experiment. He created flasks with long, thin, bent tubes attached to their necks, and boiled clear broth in them, aiming to kill any microorganisms. Some flasks had a filter in the neck, whereas others had none, but either way the tube was so narrow that dust and dirt particles were not able to penetrate, and Pasteur showed that in both these types of flask the broth did not become contaminated. Nothing grew in it unless the flasks were broken open and exposed to living organisms from outside, such as spores from dust. Therefore, microorganisms were not spontaneously generated in the broth. He won the prize.

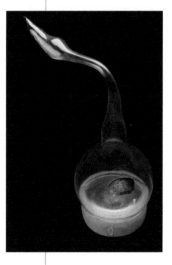

A copy of the flask Pasteur designed in 1862 to refute spontaneous generation. It was widely accepted to have won the argument although the design was not infallible, because boiling the broth did not kill all microbes.

SAVING THE WINE INDUSTRY

While he was Professor of Chemistry at
the University of Strasbourg, in the capital
of Alsace, one of France's principal
wine-growing regions, Louis Pasteur made
a discovery in 1848 that some consider
to be his most original contribution to
science. He was attempting to solve a
technical question regarding the polariza-
tion of light through tartaric acid crystals
when he realized that identical molecules
can have right- or left-handed versions,
and that those produced by living things
are always left-handed. It was a masterly
feat of observation and deduction that
boosted his reputation at any early stage of his career.

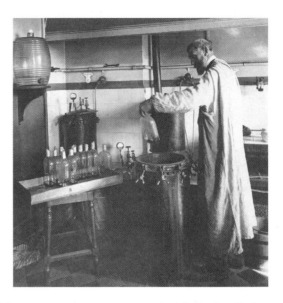

*Louis Pasteur investigating
the fermentation of wine
during his sojourn at Lille
University. He is quoted
as saying that "A bottle
of wine contains more
philosophy than all the
books in the world."*

In 1854 he was appointed Head of Science at Lille University in
northern France. Winemakers petitioned for his help in discovering
what turned wine sour, a problem that was blighting their industry.
Pasteur soon announced that the fermentation that turned sugar into
alcohol was caused by the action of microorganisms that he called
"ferments." He demonstrated that the yeast in grape skins caused
fermentation but that the process could also produce lactic acid due to
contamination by microorganisms—and that's what made wine sour.

Pasteur showed that heating beer and wine killed the bacteria that
caused them to spoil. Boiling ruined the taste—but
through experiment he found that heating to just
130°F (55°C) was enough to prolong the life of the
drink. The same principle, when applied to milk,
killed bacteria, yeasts and mold, preventing
transmission of diseases, including tuberculosis and
brucellosis, and was an important step forward in
the field of public health.

> *I am on the edge of mysteries
> and the veil is getting thinner
> and thinner ... I am often
> scolded by Madame Pasteur,
> but I console her by telling her
> that I shall lead her to fame.*
> **—LOUIS PASTEUR, LETTER, 1851**

SICKLY SILKWORMS

The next problem to which Pasteur directed his attention was that of
the silkworm diseases *pébrine* and *flacherie* that were afflicting the
silk industry in the south of France. For 6 years he studied silkworms
in his laboratory, assisted by his wife Marie, who bred them. Pasteur
worked out that the infection was being transmitted by microsporidian
parasites, and he developed a way of screening silkworm eggs so that

infected ones could be isolated and destroyed. His method is still in use today.

During the years of his silkworm research, three of Pasteur's five children died, two of typhoid and one of a tumor. In 1868 he experienced a stroke that left him partly paralyzed, but his colleagues helped to adapt his laboratory so that he could carry on working. Perhaps it was as a result of these tragedies that he turned his attention to the part micro-organisms play in human disease, spurred on by the discoveries of a physician working in a small, self-built, home laboratory near Berlin, Germany: Robert Koch.

KOCH'S DISCOVERIES

Robert Koch was a careful, methodical scientist who developed a method of producing pure cultures of bacteria on a solid medium (first gelatin, then agar jelly) and staining them so that they were visible under a microscope. His assistant Julius Petri developed the Petri dish used for this purpose. With these tools, Koch took on the daunting task of trying to match microorganisms to the diseases they caused.

He began with anthrax, a disease that was prevalent in farm animals in the area where he lived. In 1849 bacteria had been discovered in the blood of those afflicted, but Koch wanted to prove that this was the cause rather than an effect. He injected anthrax bacteria taken from a dead animal into a mouse, and as a control he injected blood from a healthy animal into another mouse. The mouse injected with anthrax developed the disease and died, whereas the control mouse was fine. Koch repeated this experiment through 20 generations of mice before reporting his conclusion in 1876.

Koch's Postulates

Koch set out four rules, or "postulates," to be applied in experiments to discover whether a microorganism is the cause of a disease:

- **A specific microorganism must be found in all creatures with the disease but not in healthy ones.**
- **The microorganism must be isolated and grown in a pure culture.**
- **When injected into a healthy host, such cultured microorganisms should cause the disease in question.**
- **The microorganisms retrieved from the creature thus infected must be identical to the original ones from which the culture was obtained.**

He later modified these postulates after finding that there can be asymptomatic carriers of diseases, such as cholera and typhoid, and that not all organisms exposed to an infectious agent will develop the disease.

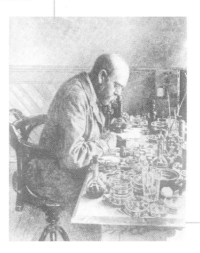

Unlike Pasteur, Robert Koch was a qualified doctor. He worked by day and carried out his groundbreaking research in his spare time, in his apartment, using a microscope given to him by his wife.

Koch would go on to discover the bacillus that causes tuberculosis (1882) and *Vibrio cholerae*, the cause of cholera (1883–4), and using his methods others would identify the bacteria causing typhus, tetanus, and plague. He was awarded a Nobel Prize for his work in 1905.

> *As soon as the right method was found, discoveries came as easily as ripe apples from a tree.*
> —ROBERT KOCH, 1882

DEVELOPING VACCINES IN THE LAB

Identifying the cause of a disease did not necessarily bring scientists closer to finding a cure, but Pasteur was determined to take the next step. He wondered if it might be possible to develop vaccines against diseases, as Jenner had for smallpox (see pages 92–95), and began to experiment with chicken cholera. In 1879, an assistant accidentally injected chickens with an old, spoiled culture of cholera virus and it caused them to develop mild symptoms of the disease but not to die. It appeared they had developed immunity from this weakened culture.

Pasteur turned his attention to anthrax and tried weakening isolated bacilli in his laboratory, first by adding antiseptic agents to his cultures and later by treating them with heat. In 1881 he injected half a group of farm animals with his weakened anthrax bacillus, then 2 weeks later he injected them all with virulent anthrax. The ones that had been vaccinated did not catch the disease, but the others did.

In 1885 an assistant of Pasteur's, Emile Roux, developed a rabies vaccine that appeared to be effective in dogs. Pasteur was nervous about trying it on humans, not least because he was not a licensed physician; but when a boy called Joseph Meister was brought to him, who had been

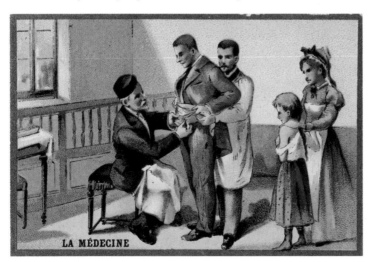

LA MÉDECINE

An illustration showing Louis Pasteur administering the rabies vaccine in his patient's abdomen. In fact, Pasteur was not allowed to give injections himself, because he was not a qualified doctor.

mauled by a rabid dog, he decided to take a chance. A physician was brought in to perform the series of 14 daily injections—and the boy did not develop rabies.

> *I am afraid that the experiments you quote,*
> *M. Pasteur, will turn against you. The world into*
> *which you wish to take us is really too fantastic.*
> —FRENCH POPULAR NEWSPAPER *LA PRESSE*, 1860

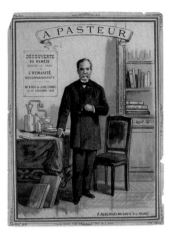

THE PASTEUR INSTITUTE

In 1887 Louis Pasteur established the Pasteur Institute in Paris to continue the study of the role of microorganisms in causing disease and the development of vaccines. He brought together scientists with different specializations and gave them state-of-the-art facilities in which to do their work, and soon the results began to flow.

The sign on the wall proclaims Pasteur to be the discoverer of a cure for rabies, a disease that was widespread in Europe in the 19th century and invariably fatal.

- Pasteur's assistants Emile Roux and Alexandre Yersin showed how the bacteria that caused the childhood killer disease diphtheria flooded the body of a person with the disease with toxins, and they developed an antitoxin to treat it.
- Yersin isolated *Yersinia pestis*, the bacterium that caused bubonic plague (see pages 56–61).
- Laveran discovered the protozoa that caused malaria (see pages 88–89).
- Jean Laigret developed a vaccine for yellow fever (see page 91).
- Calmette and Guérin developed a tuberculosis vaccine (see page 105).
- Charles Nicolle discovered how typhus is transmitted (see page 189).
- A team working at the Institute discovered the HIV virus that causes AIDS (see pages 202–205).

The Pasteur Institute continues to be in the forefront of the global battle against infectious disease to this day.

Pasteur Controversies

Before he died of a stroke in 1895, Pasteur asked his family never to show his lab notes to anyone. It was only in 1971 that they became available and researchers figured out why he had wanted them kept secret. They betray the fact that he often tidied up and even falsified his results after the fact. He lied about the method he used to produce his anthrax vaccine, saying it was oxygen-attenuated, whereas in fact he had used a sample from a colleague, Henry Toussaint, and weakened it with antiseptic. He claimed to have tested his rabies vaccine on hundreds of dogs before using it on Joseph Meister, but in fact his notes show there had been only a handful of tests. And many of his fermentation "discoveries" were the work of others.

The Snellen Eye Chart

LOCATION:	Utrecht, Netherlands
DATE:	1862
FIELD:	Ophthalmology

The scientific advances of the 18th and 19th centuries triggered progress in many fields of medicine, and one of these was ophthalmology. Physicians gained a new understanding of the anatomy of the eye, the way it worked and the diseases that could affect it. During the 18th century, eyeglasses became increasingly popular as a greater percentage of the population learned to read, but they were generally chosen on an ad hoc basis, according to the user's age. It was in the mid-19th century that Dr. Franciscus Donders devised a method of diagnosing visual acuity by getting patients to stare at a wall and report what they could see. He did not have time to devise an eye chart himself, so he left that task to his assistant, Herman Snellen.

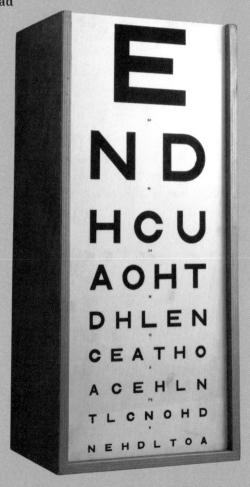

Before Kepler, all men were blind; Kepler had one eye, and Newton had two eyes.
—VOLTAIRE, QUOTED IN *VOLTAIRE'S NOTEBOOKS*, 1952

LEARNING HOW THE EYE WORKS

It took huge leaps of understanding for scientists to work out how external images make their way through the eye to the brain. Early pioneers who speculated that they traveled through the air and mingled with aqueous fluid (see page 44) were making their best guesses based on the information available. The work of Galileo and Newton paved the way for improvements in optical lenses but it was an astronomer, Johannes Kepler, working in the early 17th century, who correctly described how the eye worked. He showed that the lens and cornea are refracting media that project an inverted and reversed image onto the retina, which acts as a receiving plate. He went on to suggest that the image was later corrected "in the hollows of the brain" due to the "activity of the soul"—which, give or take the soul, is more or less correct.

Lens technology continued to improve, and in 1851 German physicist and physician Hermann von Helmholtz became famous overnight for his invention of the ophthalmoscope, making it possible to see right to the back of the eye. His *Handbook of Physiological Optics* explained his theories on the perception of depth, motion and color, and became the standard reference work for ophthalmologists. He developed a theory of accommodation to show how the pupil constricts to increase depth of field, and explained how unconscious inferences in perception (such as optical illusions or subconscious judgments) arise because of the way impressions are processed by the optic nerve. This work would influence Donders and Snellen in devising their eye test a decade later.

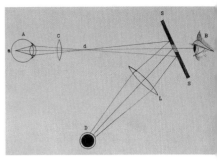

Von Helmholtz's diagram of the ophthalmoscope, which allowed physicians to see to the back of the eye. Charles Babbage in Great Britain claimed to have invented it but he did not publish his results.

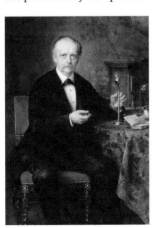

Scientist Hermann von Helmholtz mastered the disciplines of both physics and medicine. He formulated important theories on conservation of energy, thermodynamics and visual perception.

Eyeglasses

After Roger Bacon and Alexander de Spina (see page 47) developed early reading glasses, it became fashionable for men of learning to be portrayed wearing them. The earliest lenses corrected presbyopia (farsighted), then hypermetropia (a problem with focusing), and in the 16th century lenses for myopia (nearsighted) became available. Some eyeglasses had no side arms, others folded at the bridge of the nose and there were different styles and materials. Street sellers offered basketfuls of glasses and you picked the ones that seemed to work best, or the ones marked with your age, based on the assumption that everyone's eyesight deteriorated at the same rate. Only 30 percent of British men could read in the 1640s, but the number had increased to 60 percent by the mid-18th century and demand for eyeglasses increased accordingly.

TESTING VISUAL ACUITY

It was not easy to use the earliest ophthalmoscopes but for those physicians who mastered them, they provided a method of examining a wide range of eye conditions. One of the first to take advantage was Franciscus Cornelis Donders, a Dutch ophthalmologist who was universally accepted as the world's leading authority on the eye in the 1850s and 1860s. He invented the tonometer, a device that could measure intraocular pressure, enabling him to assess those at risk of glaucoma. He manufactured lenses to cure astigmatism (a condition in which the lenses fail to produce a sharp image on the retina). Doctors kept referring patients with eye problems to him and in 1858 he founded the Netherlands Hospital for Necessitous Eye Patients in Utrecht.

> *Whoever, in the pursuit of science, seeks after immediate practical utility may rest assured that he seeks in vain.*
> —HERMANN VON HELMHOLTZ, *ACADEMIC DISCOURSE*, 1862

Hermann Snellen was a young research associate to whom Donders delegated the task of devising an eye chart to test visual acuity. Previous tests had used different styles of typeface in different sizes and Donders felt that one standardized version would be helpful. Snellen's first attempt in 1861 used symbols, such as a circle, square and arrow, but there could be variation in the way patients identified these so he settled instead on letters and numbers, which he called "optotypes." All lines in his optotypes were of equal thickness, as were the white spaces between lines, and the height of each was five times the width. The original chart had seven rows of optotypes, getting progressively smaller as they went down the chart. The person taking the test stood 20 feet (6 m) away, covered one eye and read the letters, starting from the top. The smallest row that could be read indicated the visual acuity in that eye.

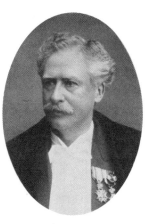

Hermann Snellen: The eye chart named after him has sold more copies in the United States than any poster, although it has now been superseded by computer-generated versions.

Snellen calculated a value for visual acuity by dividing the distance of the test from the subject by the smallest letter size they could discern. The standard became known as 20/20 vision. The system of measurement would change over the decades, and different versions of the test were used so the patient could not memorize the chart, but the principle Snellen developed is still in use today.

TREATING DISEASES OF THE EYE

The 18th and 19th centuries are often referred to as the Golden Age of Ophthalmology (actually the second one, after the earlier Islamic flowering—see pages 44–47), with many new treatments devised for age-old problems. In ancient times cataracts had been shoved aside with a needle, a technique known as couching, but that resulted in unfocused vision thereafter. The first true cataract surgery was in 1748, when Jacques Daviel extracted the opaque lens from its capsule; his patients had to be immobilized with sandbags around their heads while the incision healed, but his method had some success and cataract removal is now a common operation.

As surgery became safer, opththalmologists could treat more conditions surgically. In 1856 Berlin physician Albrecht von Graefe described an operation called a broad iridectomy to relieve the congestion of acute glaucoma, a condition that had been described by Hippocrates but which until then had meant certain blindness. In the early 20th century, Jules Gonin of Lausanne, Switzerland, developed a method of treating retinal detachment, another condition that had previously led to blindness; and in 1922 Tudor Thomas of Cardiff, Wales, inserted corneal grafts from animals. Developments in lasers (see page 199), ultrasound and microsurgery techniques throughout the 20th century mean that many of the eye conditions that blinded our ancestors can now be corrected.

Audiology

Hippocrates thought that loss of hearing was caused by changes in the direction of the wind, as well as tinnitus and head trauma. Physicians tried making loud noises in an attempt to stimulate the ears, but no real progress in treating deafness was made until the 20th century. In the 1920s, an audiometer was developed to measure hearing loss; then, after World War II, when many soldiers returned with impaired hearing either from injury, shell shock or acoustic trauma, American Raymond Carhart devised a number of hearing tests using a tuning fork and coined the term "audiology." The first electric hearing aid was produced in 1898, and now sophisticated implants within the ear can restore hearing for many.

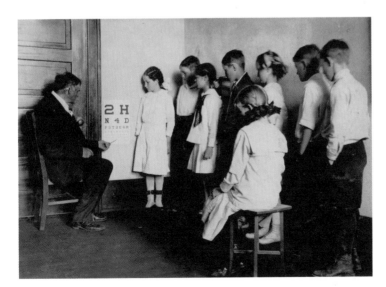

Testing the eyesight of Grade 5 pupils at school in Oklahoma, 1917, using a Snellen chart. In the 21st century, the prevalence of myopia (nearsighted) in children has doubled over the last 50 years because they spend less time playing out of doors than their predecessors.

The Red Cross Symbol

LOCATION: Geneva, Switzerland
DATE: 1861
FIELD: Battlefield medicine, humanitarian aid

In June 1859 Swiss businessman Henry Dunant toured the field after the Battle of Solferino and was horrified by the scale of suffering, with up to 40,000 men lying dead or wounded and few receiving any medical care. He came up with the idea of forming neutral societies of trained volunteers to treat those injured in battle. Medics would wear a white armband with a red cross to indicate their status. It was an idea that would greatly improve the treatment of combatants and would soon extend into peacetime as well.

In one of the Cremona hospitals, an Italian doctor had said: "We keep the good things for our friends of the Allied Army, and give our enemies the bare necessities. If they die, so much the worse!" *and he added, to excuse these barbarous words, that he had heard ... that the Austrians allowed the wounded of the Franco-Sardinian army to die uncared for.*

—HENRY DUNANT, *A MEMORY OF SOLFERINO*, 1862

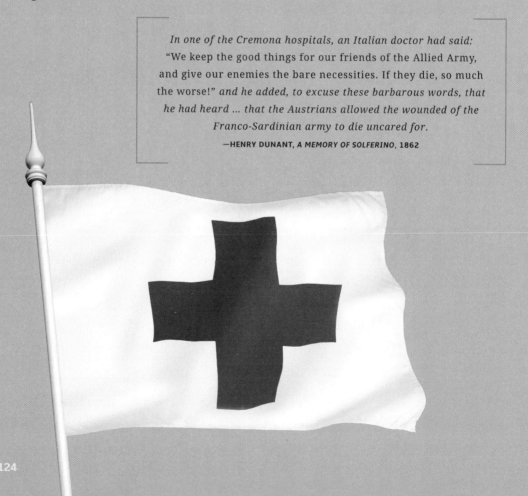

A BRIEF HISTORY OF BATTLEFIELD MEDICINE

In the time of the Roman Empire, the Roman army had well-trained military surgeons who followed the army and treated casualties from their own side. However, there was no question of treating the enemy; those unlucky enough to be captured were either slaughtered, enslaved or ransomed. Throughout the Middle Ages, prisoners of war could not expect medical treatment for their injuries, but in 1648 the Treaty of Westphalia established that at the end of hostilities they should be released without payment of ransom.

Battlefield medicine was a brutal affair, with overburdened surgeons colloquially known as "sawbones" hacking off wounded limbs in an attempt to prevent infection from setting in. Exposed tissue was cauterized with a red-hot iron or boiling oil; nevertheless, about half of all amputees died either from shock caused by blood loss, or gangrene.

During the mid-16th century, French surgeon Ambroise Paré introduced the idea of tying off bleeding arteries with ligatures, a landmark development for its time. In the early 19th century, Dominique Jean Larrey developed mobile field hospitals that could travel alongside the army, and he trained stretcher-bearers and wagon drivers to create the first ambulances, realizing that the speed with which the injured received treatment could be crucial. Larrey also taught his medical staff how to triage—in other words, to decide which cases needed help most urgently, based not on rank or nationality but on the severity of their injuries. He was a surgeon for Napoleon's army but was renowned for treating soldiers of both sides. At the Battle of Waterloo in 1815, while Larrey's men went out to collect the wounded, the Duke of Wellington ordered his troops to hold fire.

During the American Civil War of 1861–65, Dr. Jonathan Letterman created forward aid stations in which the wounded could be stabilized before they were taken to a hospital, and several medics and nurses in that war treated the wounded of both sides, as acceptance grew that this was the humane thing to do.

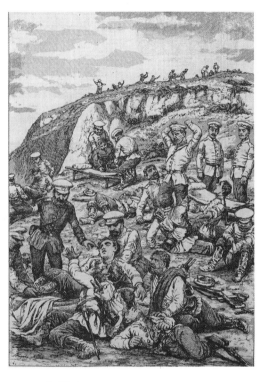

Red Cross volunteers treating casualties of the Russo-Japanese War of 1904–1905, with the red-and-white symbol on their armbands. The Russian Red Cross was founded in 1879 and the Japanese one in 1887.

Key Terms of the 1864 Geneva Convention

- Soldiers who are wounded and out of battle should be treated humanely and should not be killed or further injured.
- Wounded prisoners of war should receive medical treatment.
- Medical personnel caring for the wounded should be respected at all times.
- The identities of the dead and wounded should be noted and information passed to their own side.
- The International Red Cross (IRC) or any other impartial organization should be allowed to care for the wounded.
- The Red Cross should be adopted as an international symbol.

THE COMMITTEE OF FIVE

Henry Dunant was a Calvinist with a history of doing philanthropic work. After touring the battlefield at Solferino in 1859, he persuaded local people to help the wounded by bringing food and water as well as applying bandages and offering basic medical care. Once back in Geneva, Switzerland, he wrote a book about his experiences in which he proposed the creation of national volunteer organizations, trained in their own countries, to provide relief where needed, and he also suggested an internationally recognized charter to protect physicians working in war zones.

Henry Dunant introduced badges so that those who died in battle could be identified, campaigned for abolition of the slave trade and became joint recipient of the first Nobel Peace Prize in 1901.

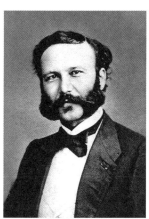

A team comprising a physician, a lawyer, an army general, and the head of the Geneva Hygiene and Health Commission got behind Dunant's ideas and held an international conference in 1863 to discuss improving medical services at the front line. One of their proposals was the adoption of the international symbol of a red cross on a white background to designate volunteers. In 1864 the first Geneva Convention was signed by 12 countries. The British Red Cross was founded in 1870, and the American one was established in 1881 by Clara Barton, who had been a popular Civil War nurse. By 1914 there were 45 national relief societies across four continents.

I have an almost complete disregard of precedent, and a faith in the possibility of something better. It irritates me to be told how things have always been done. I defy the tyranny of precedent. I go for anything new that might improve the past.

—CLARA BARTON

WARS OF THE 20TH CENTURY

During World War I, volunteer Red Cross nurses worked alongside the medical teams of combatant countries to treat those wounded in battle. Among the volunteers were American novelist Ernest Hemingway, who worked as a Red Cross ambulance driver in Italy, and English crime writer Agatha Christie, who served as a nurse. The International Red Cross (IRC) also set up an agency that created file cards for every man who was missing or taken prisoner in an effort to trace them. Seven million file cards were collected between 1914 and 1923 and 20 million letters and messages were conveyed between soldiers and their families. The IRC also reported on whether combatants were observing the terms of the Geneva Convention, and they protested vehemently when poison gas was used in the trenches—the first time chemical weapons had been used in war. After the Armistice, they helped 420,000 prisoners to return to their home countries.

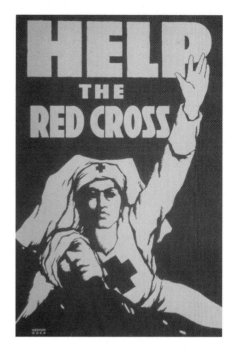

A World War I poster. There were 90,000 British Red Cross volunteers during the war and 50,000 Americans.

In 1919 the role of the IRC was extended to cover relief of crises that were not caused by war, such as natural and man-made disasters, and the Red Crescent symbol replaced the Red Cross for Muslim countries.

During World War II, combatants had their own trained medical teams, so the Red Cross's role was more concerned with the treatment of prisoners of war, the exchange of messages and tracing missing persons, although the organization did set up some auxiliary hospitals to treat the wounded of all sides. They have been involved in wars and internal conflicts ever since.

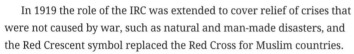

Médecins sans Frontières

In 1971 a group of French doctors formed a humanitarian, nongovernmental organization called Médecins sans Frontières (Doctors without Borders) to get medical teams to the places in the world where they are most needed. They were moved to act by the horrors of the Nigerian Civil War of 1967–70, in which Biafrans were besieged in desperate conditions. MSF's first mission was to help victims of a 1972 earthquake in Nicaragua, and they developed lightning-response teams that could be jetted into emergencies. Since then, they have become involved in providing vaccination programs, water purification and sanitation plans, as well as feeding centers in areas where there is malnutrition. By 2015 they had 30,000 healthcare workers in more than 70 countries.

Joseph Lister's Donkey Engine

LOCATION:	Glasgow, Scotland
DATE:	1871
FIELD:	Surgery

By the mid-19th century, many physicians were thinking of abandoning surgery, because post-operative infection (known as "ward fever") caused such high death rates. It was still believed that infection came from miasma, and several hospitals aired their wards daily to try to prevent it. The airings did little good, however, when surgeons did not wash their hands or clean their instruments between patients, carrying infected pus from one to the next. Joseph Lister read about Louis Pasteur's theories on fermentation and wondered if microorganisms might cause infection in wounds in the same way as they ruined wine. It was an ingenious deduction and his introduction of antisepsis would revolutionize surgery.

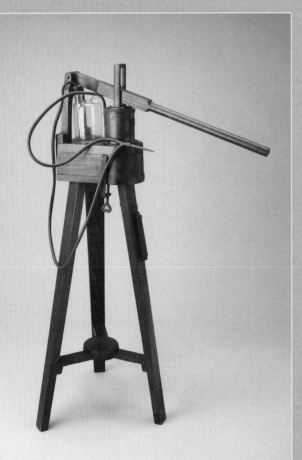

> When almost every wound was foul with suppuration, it seemed natural ... to postpone the cleansing of hands and instruments until the process of dressings and probings had been finished.
>
> —A DOCTOR SPEAKING IN THE 1860S, QUOTED IN NANCY DUIN AND JENNY SUTCLIFFE, *A HISTORY OF MEDICINE*, 1992

LAUDABLE PUS

Early 19th-century surgeons were proud to wear heavily stained gowns and operate in blood-soaked operating rooms with what was called "that good old surgical stink," because it demonstrated their wealth of experience. There was no attempt to clean bed linen, lab coats and instruments between patients, and it was believed that "laudable pus," first described by Galen, eliminated unhealthy humors. The mortality rate in 1860s hospitals was about 12 percent of all patients, and close to 50 percent for amputees.

In 1843 Oliver Wendell Holmes published an article in the *New England Journal of Medicine* suggesting that puerperal fever was spread on contact, and noting cases of doctors who had died of it after performing autopsies on victims. He was not taken seriously, however, and his article was not widely publicized. In Vienna, Austria, Ignaz Semmelweis (see page 115) insisted that after performing an operation doctors should wash their hands in calcium chloride before visiting a new patient; deaths on his wards fell from 12 percent to 1 percent, but his findings were ignored by the medical establishment.

Florence Nightingale's *Notes on Nursing*, published in 1859, advocated fresh air and sunlight, pure water, cleanliness and adequate sanitation in hospital wards, based on her experiences in the Crimean War, where "ward fever" was rife (see pages 110–13). She did not know exactly why cleanliness was effective but she was thinking along roughly the right lines.

Gangrene

Gangrene is necrosis (cell death) caused when there is insufficient blood supply to an area of tissue, most often at the extremities. In wet gangrene, the most common type in hospitals in the 19th century, open wounds are invaded by putrefying bacteria, causing the tissues to swell up and give off a fetid smell. The toxic products of putrefaction are absorbed into the blood, causing sepsis and eventual death, and the only treatment is amputation above the affected area. Gas gangrene is caused by bacteria from soil infecting a wound, and was common among soldiers injured in the trenches during World War I. It produces gas within the tissues and can rapidly lead to sepsis. Dry gangrene is often a side effect of diabetes or peripheral artery disease, whereas necrotizing fasciitis, the so-called "flesh-eating disease," is a rare infection caused by streptococcal bacteria.

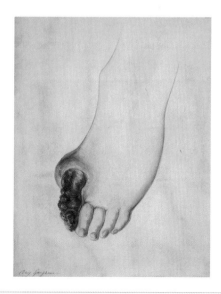

Dry gangrene of the big toe: The cells have died as a result of insufficient blood reaching them and eventually the digit will fall off.

THE DONKEY ENGINE

As a young physician Joseph Lister spent many years studying inflammation and concluded that it was not a disease in itself but a response to infection that rendered tissues useless. He postulated that a similar process to Pasteur's fermentation (see page 116) might be causing infection in open wounds. At the time, carbolic acid was used to treat sewage spread in fields, and it appeared to cause no ill effects in cattle that fed there later, so Lister concluded it should be safe to use on wounds. In March 1865 he began to perform antiseptic operations with his instruments and hands cleaned in carbolic acid and the wound dressed with a bandage soaked in 5 percent carbolic acid solution. Soon the rate of postoperative infection in his patients was dropping.

In August 1865, a young boy called James Greenlees was brought to Lister. He had been run over by a cart that resulted in a compound fracture of his leg. In a compound fracture, the broken end of the bone pierces the skin. Normally such fractures required amputation to prevent the spread of infection, but Lister washed the wound with carbolic acid and flaxseed oil, then dressed it in aluminum foil. When he checked after a few days, there was no sign of infection, and 6 weeks later the boy was able to walk out of the hospital, his leg saved. Lister published his results in the leading medical journal, *The Lancet*, in 1867, but the reception among doctors was critical and nurses complained about the extra work it would entail for them if they had to keep operating rooms spotlessly clean.

Undeterred, Lister continued to develop his methods. He invented a machine known as the donkey engine, which could spray a fine mist of carbolic solution into the air in the operating room. The solution was placed in a bottle mounted on a tripod and an assistant pumped the long handle. In 1872–73 the carbolic solution was changed for a steam spray because carbolic acid irritated the lungs. The results were a clear vindication of his method: only 2 percent of Lister's surgical patients were dying.

Joseph Lister's donkey engine in use during surgery. He insisted that all the surgeons with whom he worked should wash their hands before and after operations in a solution of 5 percent carbolic acid, and clean their instruments in the same.

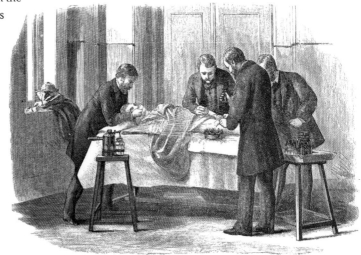

> *Previous to its introduction, the 2 large wards in which most of my cases of accident and of operation are treated were amongst the unhealthiest in the whole of [the] surgical division at the Glasgow Royal Infirmary ... but since the antiseptic treatment has been brought into full operation, ... my wards ... have completely changed their character; so that during the last 9 months not a single instance of pyaemia, hospital gangrene or erysipelas has occurred in them.*

—JOSEPH LISTER, ADDRESSING THE BRITISH MEDICAL ASSOCIATION, 1867

LISTER'S LEGACY

Lister devised many other improvements in surgery: he replaced the silk that had previously been used for surgical ligatures with catgut, which would be naturally absorbed by the body and did not cause irritation; he introduced nonporous materials for the handles of surgical instruments; and he was responsible for pioneering several new operations, including a method of repairing kneecaps with metal wire.

After Queen Victoria allowed the use of carbolic spray when she had a minor operation in 1871, it began to catch on, and once antiseptic practice was widely adopted, the death rate in hospitals fell to an average of 5 percent—a staggering improvement on the earlier 12 percent. Compound fractures no longer required amputation of the limb, and abdominal and chest surgery were now possible.

German surgeon Ernst von Bergmann introduced heat sterilization of surgical instruments in 1886, and in 1891 he pioneered aseptic surgery (in which operating rooms are sterile environments). During the 1880s Polish surgeon Jan Mikulicz-Radecki, a great believer in Lister's techniques, created a surgical mask and used medical gloves during operations. New York surgeon William Halsted introduced many modern surgical principles, and pioneered a number of new operations, including the mastectomy for breast cancer.

Halsted's Principles for Surgery

In 1877, when his New York hospital refused to invest in a sterile operating room, William Halsted spent $10,000 of his own money creating one in a tent in the grounds of the hospital. In 1881, when his sister had a hemorrhage after giving birth, he saved her life by transfusing some of his own blood; then the following year he performed emergency gallbladder surgery on his mother, operating on her kitchen table after dipping his hands and his instruments into carbolic acid. The surgical principles he proposed included the gentle handling of body tissues, scrupulous control over blood loss, sterile conditions in the operating room, surgeons wearing gowns and rubber gloves, and tension-free closure of wounds.

The X-ray Machine

LOCATION:	Würzburg, Germany
DATE:	1895
FIELD:	Radiology, oncology

Physicist Wilhelm Röntgen was studying electricity when he accidentally discovered a new kind of ray that allowed him to see bones beneath the skin. He had no idea what it was and named it the x-ray, since x was the mathematical symbol for a variable of unknown quantity. Word spread rapidly and soon everyone was thinking of applications for this mysterious ray, with generals taking x-ray machines into battle and fairgrounds inviting visitors to view images of their own bones. A few weeks after Röntgen's discovery, Henri Becquerel found that natural rays were emitted by uranium salts, and Pierre and Marie Curie later christened them "radioactivity." Between them they were taking medical science from the 19th into the 20th century.

> *We are sick of the Röntgen rays … you can see other people's bones with the naked eye, and also see through 8 inches of solid wood. On the revolting indecency of this there is no need to dwell … perhaps the best thing would be for all civilized nations to combine: to burn all works on the Röntgen rays, to execute all the discoverers.*
> —PALL MALL GAZETTE, 1896

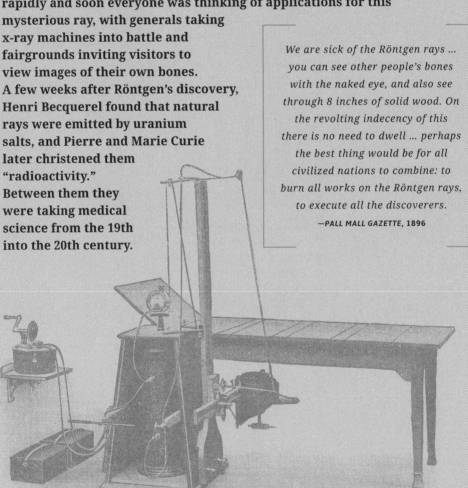

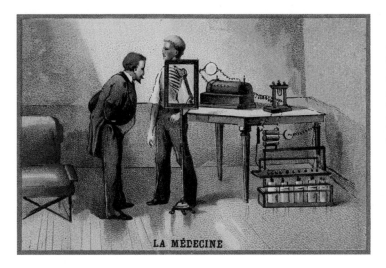

Illustration of Röntgen peering into an x-ray machine. He didn't know what the mysterious rays he discovered in 1895 actually were, but 17 years later Max von Laue found they were short-wavelength electromagnetic waves.

THE BIRTH OF THE X-RAY

Huge scientific advances in the early 19th century allowed physicists Alessandro Volta, André-Marie Ampère and Michael Faraday to harness and explore the properties of electricity, and in 1834 William Henry Fox Talbot produced the first photographic image by placing objects onto paper brushed with light-sensitive silver chloride, which he then exposed to sunlight. Improvements to vacuum technology in the 1850s allowed English physicist William Crookes to produce a partly evacuated tube in which a high voltage could be passed between two electrodes, allowing the study of cathode rays. Wilhelm Röntgen, Professor of Physics at Würzburg University in Germany, was exploring the path of such rays in a Crookes tube covered in black cardboard to block out light, when he noticed that a screen covered in phosphorescent material on his workbench was glowing with a faint green light. He deduced that rays were somehow penetrating the cardboard.

For the next 6 weeks, Röntgen experimented with these rays and found they penetrated wood, paper, the walls of his laboratory and all kinds of other substances—but not lead. When he held up a lead object between the Crooke's tube and the phosphorescent screen, he could see the outline

Unusual Uses of X-rays

The 20 million visitors who attended the St. Louis World Fair in 1904 were offered the chance to see their own bones in an x-ray machine, and these soon became common fairground attractions. Well-bred ladies were alarmed at the idea of machines that could see beneath their clothing, and a London firm rushed to create a new type of underwear they claimed could not be penetrated by x-rays. In New York there was a press report that the College of Physicians was using x-rays to print anatomical drawings into the brains of medical students, and a farmer in Ohio claimed he had used x-rays to turn base metal to gold.

In the 21st century, x-rays have many nonmedical uses, including the scanning of paintings to see what lies beneath the surface, checking that airport passengers are not carrying weapons and finding fingerprints at crime scenes that would otherwise have been missed.

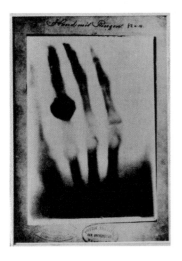

of the lead and also the bones of his hand. He got his wife to hold her hand over a photographic plate while he directed the rays at it, and created an image in which the bones of her hand and the outline of her wedding ring were clearly visible. He published his results and they were eagerly taken up by the scientific community and the public at large. At last it was possible to see what was happening inside the body without actually cutting it open.

Röntgen's wife's hand, the first-ever x-ray, which was taken in 1895. "I have seen my death!" she cried, on being shown the image.

X-RAYS IN HEALTH CARE

In 1896, Glasgow Royal Infirmary in Scotland opened one of the first radiology departments, where Dr. John Macintyre took images of a penny lodged in the throat of a child and kidney stones in a patient. Dr. John Hall-Edwards in Birmingham, England, radiographed the wrist of a maid and located a needle embedded inside, and he was the first to produce a radiograph of the spine. Lord Kitchener took a mobile x-ray machine to the Sudan in 1898, and after the Battle of Omdurman it was used to diagnose broken bones and locate bullets embedded in the flesh of wounded soldiers. X-ray machines, such as the Omniscope, were invented in which patients could be moved around and x-rayed from different angles.

In 1913 German surgeon Albert Salomon studied 3,000 breast x-rays, and found it was possible to distinguish cancerous from noncancerous tumors by looking for tiny deposits of calcium. Mammograms are now routinely offered to women aged over 50.

Researchers began looking for a medium that would allow them to see soft tissues as well as hard. In 1896 Walter B. Cannon of Harvard University had shown that when laboratory animals were given a dose of bismuth salts, their intestines were visible on a fluorescent screen. In 1904 the first human patients were given barium sulfate, and x-rays showed their intestines; it was the first "barium meal," a technique that is still used today.

The dose of radiation used in early x-rays was about 1,500 times greater than that used in the 21st century and the exposure needed to get an image was up to 90 minutes. Radiologists were soon noticing burns on their hands, and some began to wonder whether these new rays

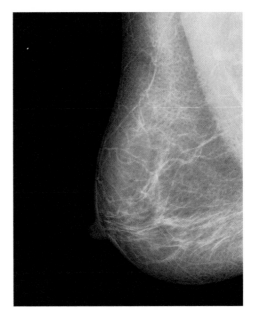

could be of use in eradicating cancerous tumors. In 1896 Emil Grubbe, a Chicago medical student, persuaded his professor to let him irradiate a woman named Rose Lee, who had advanced breast cancer. She seemed to benefit from it, and the practice became widespread. Georg Perthes in Bonn, Germany, used radiology to treat skin cancer and warts as well as breast cancer, with encouraging results.

Side effects of radiation were noted as early as 1902, when A. Frieben, a German radiologist, reported the development of skin cancer in a technician who had been working with x-rays; but the effects were cumulative and long-term, and it would be decades before these early pioneers began to succumb to cancers and radiation sickness.

RADIOACTIVITY

Weeks after Röntgen's discovery of x-rays, French physicist Henri Becquerel wondered whether phosphorescent uranium salts placed on a photographic plate would emit x-ray-style radiation when exposed to sunlight. He set up the experiment before realizing that it was a dull day, so he wrapped the plate and put it away in a drawer. When he returned he found the plate was darkened in the spot where the salts had been, and concluded that the uranium must have emitted rays without the application of any external energy source. He had discovered natural radioactivity.

In 1897 Polish student Marie Curie was doing a doctoral thesis on uranium rays at the Sorbonne School of Physics and Chemistry in Paris, France, where her husband Pierre taught. Using an electrometer developed by Pierre, she found that pitchblende (a form of uranium oxide) was four times as radioactive as uranium itself. Pierre joined her as they began the search for even more radioactive substances, by refining pitchblende and chalcolite. In 1898 they produced a substance 330 times as radioactive as uranium and named it polonium, after Marie's native Poland. For the next 3 years they continued this painstaking work until they

Radiation Casualties

Dozens of early radiologists died as a result of their exposure to high doses of radiation. Clarence Dally, who worked in Thomas Edison's lab, died of metastatic carcinoma in 1904 at the age of 39. Henri Becquerel developed serious burns on his skin that may have contributed to his sudden death in 1908. Fritz Giesel, who helped establish the first dental x-ray lab, died of metastatic carcinoma in 1927. Marie Curie died in 1934 of aplastic anemia, an illness brought on by prolonged exposure to radium. And Emil Grubbe had 83 cancer operations and became sterile before dying of cancer in 1960, completely aware that his work had caused it: "Like many of the early pioneers, I too, will die a victim of natural science, a martyr to the x-rays," he said.

Nothing in life is to be feared, it is only to be understood. Now is the time to understand more, so that we may fear less.
—MARIE CURIE, *RADIOACTIVE SUBSTANCES*, 1903

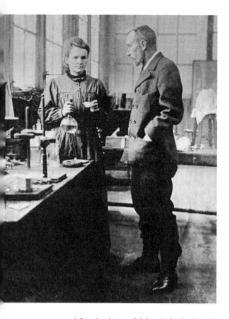

had isolated one tenth of a gram of highly radioactive pure radium. In 1901 Henri Becquerel found that his skin was burned and severely inflamed after he had carried a vial of radium in his vest pocket. Marie and Pierre Curie explored this side effect and found that when exposed to radium, cancer cells were destroyed at a faster rate than the surrounding cells. It was an important breakthrough.

Marie and Pierre Curie: Pierre was killed by a horse-drawn cart in 1906, but Marie continued their research. She spent the Nobel Prize money she received buying field ambulances equipped with x-ray machines for use during World War I and establishing x-ray departments in 200 hospitals.

RADIATION THERAPY

Radium could be applied to patients in ways that x-rays could not. Mixed with air, it could be inhaled to treat diseases of the lungs, such as tuberculosis. Radium salts could be added to baths to treat arthritis, gout and neuralgia. Small tubes containing radium could be attached to the skin at the exact site of a tumor (a procedure known as brachytherapy), or it could be condensed and mixed with glycerin or lanolin to be used as a cream for skin cancers. Dilute solutions of radium salts were even taken internally. x-rays were still used for larger areas of cancer, but radium could target soft-tissue cancers in a specific localized area.

Marie Curie appointed Claudius Regaud to research the medical effects of radiology, and he found that it was better tolerated and more successful if modest doses were given over several weeks instead of one large dose, a process known as "fractionation." French radiologist Henri Coutard pioneered the use of fractionated radiation therapy for a wide range of tumors and achieved particularly impressive results in treating laryngeal cancer. However, early radiation-therapy machines could not penetrate enough to affect deep cancers without damaging the skin and overlying tissues.

In the 1950s a linear accelerator was developed that produced high-energy, deeply penetrating beams that could for the first time

Gordon Isaacs, the first patient treated with the linear accelerator for cancer of the eye, seen here with the machine in 1957.

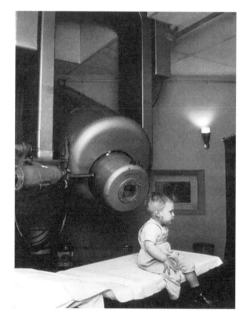

target deep tumors. The first patient treated with it was a child with cancer of the eye, and it was a complete success, with the patient retaining good vision 40 years later. By the late 1980s computerized tomographic imaging (see page 195) improved the delivery of radiation therapy and minimized damage to surrounding cells; and IMRT (intensity-modulated radiation therapy) now allows the dose to be targeted exactly in three dimensions, while a combined MRI scanner (see pages 194–97) and radiation-therapy machine allows radiologists to see the tumor as they treat it.

CANCER TREATMENT IN THE 21ST CENTURY

Nowadays, cancer treatment normally involves a cocktail of surgery, chemotherapy and radiation therapy. An understanding of the role of hormones in feeding some cancers has led to medicines such as tamoxifen that can suppress their effects. Other cancer drugs stimulate interferons, the body's natural cancer-fighting substances, and it seems certain that more sophisticated pharmacology aligned with gene therapy (see pages 183–84), microsurgery (see page 199) and nanotechnology (see page 201) will greatly reduce mortality in the future.

Public health campaigns, such as the one about the dangers of smoking (see page 188), have played a huge role in reducing deaths from cancer, and new research appears regularly about the anticancer benefits of some substances and the carcinogenic qualities of others. Research is currently ongoing to discover a pill that could prevent certain cancers altogether, and there are promising results with aspirin (see pages 138–41).

History of Cancer Treatment

Cancer was recognized by the ancient Greeks. Galen thought it was caused by too much blood, but the only treatment he proposed was prompt excision of the whole cancerous mass. During the 17th century, the involvement of the lymph nodes in cancer was recognized, and in the 18th century Marie-François Bichat proposed that cancers were an overgrowth of tissues. It was in the 19th century that Rudolf Virchow realized that uncontrolled cell division caused the growth of tumors, but he suggested this was due to "irritation of the cells." Chemotherapy was first tried in 1865 when potassium arsenite was used to treat leukemia, but it was not until the 1940s that the first truly effective medications were found, based on the deadly mustard gas used as a weapon during World War I.

Every great advance in science has issued from a new audacity of the imagination.
—U.S. PHILOSOPHER JOHN DEWEY,
THE QUEST FOR CERTAINTY, 1929

Bayer Aspirin

LOCATION:	Barmen, Germany
DATE:	1895
FIELD:	Pharmacology

Physicians throughout history have sought ways of alleviating chronic pain, such as that caused by arthritis, toothache and headaches. All kinds of methods have been tried, from trepanation to acupuncture and herbal remedies. Salicylic acid, found in willow bark, meadowsweet and a number of other plants, was long known to have pain-relieving qualities, but it caused severe gastric irritation. In 1895, when the head of research at the German Bayer Company asked Felix Hoffmann to find a type of salicylic acid without side effects, he had an extra-strong motivation, because his father was crippled by arthritis. The medicine he created, named aspirin, would become the first mass-market pain-killer.

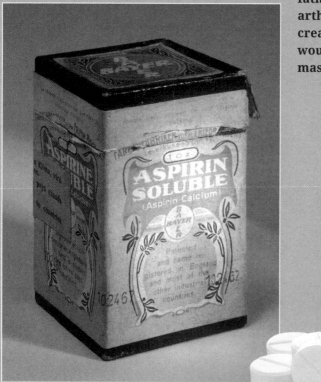

EARLY ADVOCATES OF WILLOW BARK

In Neolithic times, when it was believed that pain was caused by evil spirits, trepanation (see pages 8–11) may have been performed in an effort to relieve it. Ancient Egyptians laid electric eels found in the Nile River across the body in an attempt to alleviate pain. The ancient Chinese (see pages 22–25) developed acupuncture, whereas the Inca chewed coca leaves (from which cocaine is derived). American Indians chewed willow bark, and both Hippocrates and Dioscorides recommended it for the relief of fever, inflammation and pain.

In 1763 the Reverend Edward Stone, from Oxfordshire in England, found that chewing the bark of the white willow (*Salix alba*) helped to relieve ague, a fever associated with malaria. He set up a trial of 50 people with ague, who all agreed with him about the benefits, but when he wrote to the President of the Royal Society with his findings the letter was ignored.

During the 1820s, pharmacists succeeded in extracting salicylic acid from the leaves of meadowsweet (*Filipendula ulmaria*), but it caused such irritation to the stomach, with vomiting, nausea, bleeding and ulcers, that only those in the most severe pain were prepared to tolerate the side effects. It wasn't until the 1890s that Arthur Eichengrün at the German pharmaceutical company Bayer asked Felix Hoffmann to work on it.

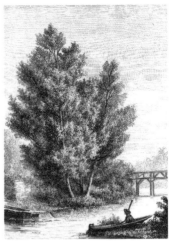

White willow (Salix alba) and, below, its medicinal bark: Hippocrates, Galen and Pliny the Elder all mentioned that the leaves and bark could ease pain and reduce fever.

The Placebo Effect

Various clinical trials between the 1970s and 1990s established that patients can experience substantial reduction in pain when they expect that a treatment will offer pain relief, even if it has no specific physiological analgesic action. This is known as the placebo effect (from the Latin *placebo*, "I will please"). In a 2004 study at Columbia University, in which electric shocks or heat patches were applied to volunteers' skin, they reported 70 percent less pain after application of a placebo skin cream, and MRI scans confirmed that the pain centers in the brain fired off fewer signals. Conversely, if patients view a treatment as harmful, they are more likely to report negative effects—the *nocebo* ("I will harm") effect.

BAYER'S BREAKTHROUGH

Hoffmann found that if he converted salicylic acid into the compound acetylsalicylic acid, the body could absorb it without significant side effects. He took some home for his arthritic father to try, and the old man had his first pain-free night in years. Hoffmann's colleague Heinrich Dreser worked out that acetylsalicylic acid broke down in the blood, thus avoiding the gastric problems. Bayer named the new medicine aspirin—the a from acetyl and the spir from spirea, an older botanical name for meadowsweet—and patented it on March 6, 1899.

It appeared in pill form in 1900, and in 1915 it became available to the public without prescription. It was the first over-the-counter mass-market medicine, and proved an enormous success for Bayer.

In 1914, when World War I began, the British government no longer wanted to pay a German company for supplies of aspirin. They announced a competition with prize money of £20,000 for any pharmacist who could come up with a new formula that would get around the patent, and the Australian premier added £5,000 to the kitty. Australian pharmacist George Nicholas managed to produce pure acetylsalicylic acid in a makeshift laboratory, despite nearly blinding himself in an ether explosion. In 1917 he registered it under the trade name Aspro and it was soon selling in many countries, including Great Britain and Australia. In America, Bayer sold their patent to Sterling for an unprecedented $3 million, and Bayer aspirin continued to be the market leader there.

Everyone knew aspirin worked, but it was only in 1971 that British pharmacologist John Robert Vane discovered how. He found that it was prostaglandins (compounds with hormonelike effects) released at the site of an injury that cause the pain response, and observed that aspirin binds to the enzyme that produces prostaglandin. Although high doses of aspirin could still irritate the stomach, it truly was a miracle drug. In the following decades, it was found to have other uses besides treating pain and inflammation, with proven efficacy in preventing coronary artery disease, heart attack and stroke. It may also limit the development and growth of prostate, colon, pancreatic and lung cancers—something Felix Hoffmann never suspected.

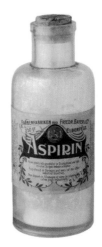

One of the first aspirin bottles, 1899. By the 1950s aspirin would enter the Guinness Book of Records as the world's most purchased painkiller.

The Physicians' Health Study

In the 1980s Harvard epidemiologist Charles Hennekens ran a major clinical trial to investigate the benefits of aspirin use. He enrolled 22,071 male physicians to take a pill daily for 10 years, without knowing whether they were taking aspirin or a placebo. After 5 years, it was clear that the aspirin group had a 44 percent lower risk of heart attack and it was decided that the placebo group should be allowed to take aspirin, too. Hennekens also discovered that those given an aspirin within 24 hours of a heart attack or stroke had their risk of a second attack reduced by one quarter, because of the way that aspirin hinders the blood platelets from forming clots.

OTHER TYPES OF PAIN-KILLERS

- Aspirin is one of a group of nonsteroidal anti-inflammatory drugs (NSAIDs) that also includes ibuprofen, indomethacin and naproxen. These medicines reduce fever, inflammation and pain, and are especially good for relieving arthritis pain.

- Acetaminophen (paracetamol) was first manufactured in 1873 but was not used medically until the 1950s, when it went on sale as Tylenol in the United States and Panadol in Britain. Its ability to block pain receptors made it ideal for treating headaches, colds and flu.

- Narcotic analgesics, including codeine and morphine, are still prescribed to decrease pain, but they have many of the side effects common to the opiates of old, including constipation and drowsiness.

- Anticonvulsants are often used for neuropathic pain, such as trigeminal neuralgia, because of their ability to stabilize nerve cells.

- Muscle relaxants, such as Valium (diazepam), can be prescribed for lower back pain and spinal cord injury.

Nerve block injections and corticosteroid creams are among other methods of pain relief, but modern pain management clinics may also refer patients for acupuncture (see page 25), which may block transmission of pain impulses, or TENS machines, which use gentle electrical stimulation—just like those electric eels used by the ancient Egyptians.

> *Researchers have found that placebo treatments— interventions with no active drug ingredients—can stimulate real physiological responses, from changes in heart rate and blood pressure to chemical activity in the brain in cases involving pain, depression, anxiety, fatigue and even some symptoms of Parkinson's.*
> —CARA FEINBERG,
> *HARVARD MAGAZINE*, 2013

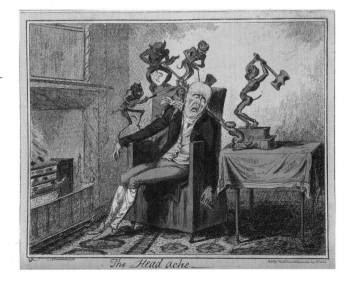

The Headache, *by Isaac Cruikshank, ca. 1830. American poet Emily Dickinson, who experienced migraines, described the sensation in her poem "Funeral in my brain" as feeling like mourners treading around in "boots of lead."*

Sigmund Freud's Couch

LOCATION: Vienna, Austria
DATE: Early 20th century
FIELD: Psychiatry, psychoanalysis

Unexpressed emotions will never die. They are buried alive and will come forth later in uglier ways.
—SIGMUND FREUD

Medical advances moved rapidly from the 16th through the 19th centuries, but research into mental health did not keep pace. Up to the Middle Ages and well beyond, the mentally ill were thought to be possessed by demons or evil spirits and were subjected to violent exorcisms and painful treatments designed to purify them. The first lunatic asylum was opened in Valencia, Spain, in 1406, and other countries followed suit, creating institutions where inmates were treated as animals to be subdued. The straitjacket was introduced in the 19th century, as well as a revolving chair designed to shake patients out of their malady. This is why it was considered radical in 1905 when Sigmund Freud first set out his ideas on curing the mentally ill simply by listening to what they had to say.

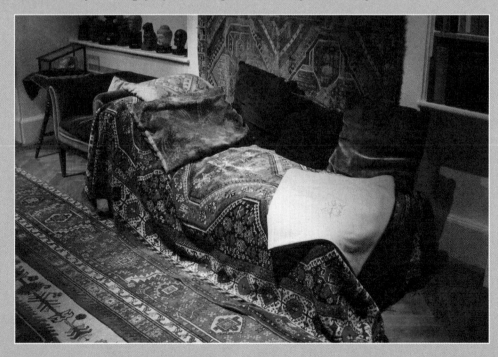

THE EFFICACY OF KINDNESS

In 1792, Philippe Pinel, the superintendent of the Bicêtre asylum in Paris, France, demonstrated that restraining mentally ill patients made their condition worse, whereas letting them wander free and treating them with kindness could even lead to some being cured. In England his thinking chimed with observations of King George III, who experienced episodes of severe mental illness now thought to have been caused by hereditary porphyria. In York, England, a Quaker family opened the first private asylum in the 1790s in which restraint was not used, and it proved highly successful In Boston, Massachusetts, Dorothea Dix campaigned relentlessly in the 1840s for better treatment of the mentally ill. However, the attitude that "lunatics" could somehow be shocked out of their lunacy remained, and they were still treated as animals. In Victorian London, citizens paid a penny and lined up to stare at the most violent inmates of Bedlam (officially Bethlem Royal Hospital).

By the second half of the 19th century, French neurologist Jean-Martin Charcot was proposing that hysteria might have a neurological basis. He treated his patients with hypnosis, magnets, and the application of various metals in an attempt to cure the physical root cause. Among those who came to study his work was a young medical student named Sigmund Freud.

On his return to Vienna, Austria, Freud became fascinated by a patient of his colleague Dr. Josef Breuer, a woman known as "Anna O." When Breuer used hypnosis on Anna O., he became convinced that her many symptoms, including memory loss, problems with speech and sight, disorientation, nausea and limb paralysis, were linked to traumas she had experienced in the past. Freud was persuaded by this, and in 1896 he opened his own private medical practice specializing in nervous disorders.

Mesmerism

In the second half of the 18th century, German doctor Franz Mesmer became famous for his claims that he could restore health by enlisting a natural force known as "animal magnetism." At his Magnetic Institute in Paris, France, clients stood around a chemical bath holding onto an iron ring, while the doctor moved his hands over and around them. Many fell into a kind of trance, and when they came around, they felt much better. The popularity of "mesmerism" spread, but an Académie des Sciences investigation pronounced that any results came from the power of the imagination. After observing animal magnetism, Scottish scientist James Braid proposed that the patient's suggestibility while in a trance could be useful in treating nervous disorders, and went on to develop hypnotism.

An engraving of 1794 showing the induction of a hypnotic trance in a female patient.

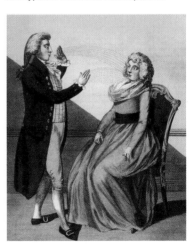

THEORY OF THE SUBCONSCIOUS

Freud tried hypnosis on his patients but soon decided it didn't work and opted instead for a technique he called "free association." Patients were invited to lie on his couch with their eyes closed and talk randomly about whatever came into their minds, prompted by occasional questions or observations from the doctor. Freud searched in these rambling monologues for associations that would reveal the inner workings of the patient's mind and lead to the root cause of their ailment. Sometimes these would become apparent through a misspoken word, which became known as the "Freudian slip."

In order to augment his understanding of the inner workings of the brain, Freud began the long process of self-analysis by recording and interpreting his dreams. In his widely noticed 1905 book *The Interpretation of Dreams*, he argued that all dreams feature a kind of wish-fulfillment fantasy. Anxieties and fears appear jumbled up and rearranged, with symbols representing subjects in everyday life. By deconstructing these dreams, Freud claimed he could open a window into the inner life.

Based on his work with early patients, Freud surmised that unconscious memories of sexual molestation during early childhood were a prime cause of neuroses. From there he developed his controversial Oedipus complex theory, which suggested that we grow up subconsciously attracted to our opposite-sex parent and confused by our repression of this memory. Only by uncovering these repressed thoughts in therapy can we cure ourselves. However, when Freud suggested to a patient by the name of Ida Bauer, whom he called Dora, that the reason why she kept losing her voice was because she had repressed her desire for her father, she walked out of treatment.

Famous Patients

Freud claimed that his patient Dora felt jealous of her father's relationship with a family friend. When she told him of a dream in which her father refused to let her rescue her jewel case from a fire, he suggested that the jewel case represented her virginity. Rat Man was the name given by Freud to a patient who had obsessive thoughts about rats, a fear that Freud thought represented guilt about his anal sexual fantasies. Wolf Man was a Russian patient who experienced depression; his nickname came from a dream about a tree full of white wolves, which Freud believed referred to a childhood experience in which he witnessed his parents having sex.

Freud called dreams "The Royal Road to the Unconscious," because the mind's internal censor is less alert than in waking hours, allowing buried trauma to emerge.

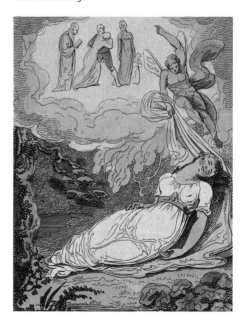

THE ID, THE EGO AND THE SUPEREGO

Between 1888 and 1939 Freud published 24 books expanding on different aspects of his theories. Perhaps the most significant part of his work lies in his description of the three parts of the human psyche. The id is the impulsive, pleasure-seeking part that seeks instant gratification of desires, such as sex or aggression. The superego is the part that understands the moral values of society and incorporates the conscience, which makes us feel guilty if we do wrong, and our image of the ideal self to which we aspire. The third part, the ego, develops to mediate between the id and the superego and make decisions about how to behave. Freud argued that a newborn child is all id and gradually develops ego and superego through what it learns from its parents and society. He explained that neuroses and anxieties arise from conflict between these three parts, most of which are subconscious.

Freudian theory attracted a lot of attention and in 1910 the International Psychoanalytic Association was founded in Vienna. The first congress was attended by 42 physicians, but soon there were rifts between them. Alfred Adler rejected Freud's emphasis on sex and claimed that humans are primarily motivated by a sense of powerlessness and feelings of inferiority. Although a founder member of the group, he broke away to form his own branch of analysis based on personality. Karl Jung placed emphasis on what he called the "collective unconscious" that was shared by societies. It derived from our ancestors and consisted of spiritual, creative energies and archetypes that shaped our thoughts and desires. In Russia, Anton Pavlov was using dogs and rats to demonstrate the power of conditioning and arguing that human behavior is similarly the result of conditioning. French psychoanalyst Jacques Lacan focused on the importance of language and discourse. But Freud was the acknowledged inventor of the new philosophy of psychoanalysis.

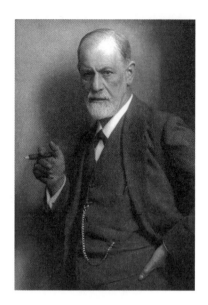

Sigmund Freud: his patients lay on the famous couch while he sat out of sight to ensure no eye contact between them, which might inhibit free association.

Transference

Freud described the process of transference during analysis, whereby patients subconsciously transfer their own feelings about a parent or other figure for whom they have repressed desires to the analyst. Sometimes it caused clients to think they had fallen in love with their analyst, whereas at other times it made them hostile and uncooperative in the process, but in either case the unconscious was revealed, so Freud considered it an important analytic tool. He also described the process of countertransference, in which an analyst began to have emotional feelings toward the client.

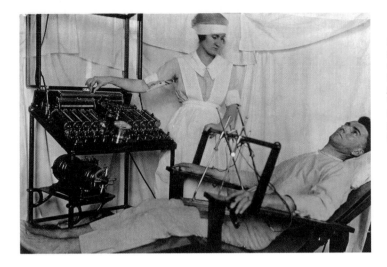

The Bergonic chair was used in the early 20th century to administer mild electric shocks to patients experiencing "psycho-neuroses." It was not until the 1930s that electricity was used to induce seizures.

SHOCK TREATMENTS

By the 1930s many were losing patience with Freud's talking cure; it took too long and often didn't work. Medical scientists began to devise more physically intrusive methods in an attempt to heal the mentally ill. In 1933 German physician Manfred Sakel injected a schizophrenic patient with enough insulin to send him into a coma, hoping the shock would cure him. (Sakel claimed his method was successful in 88 percent of patients, but scientific analysis of his results found no real benefits and some fatalities.) This was followed in 1938 by the development of electroconvulsive therapy (ECT) by two Italians, Ugo Cerletti and Lucio Bini. The idea of giving electric shocks to the brain was terrifying for patients, and its reputation was not enhanced by tales of bones broken due to the violence of the convulsions and the smell of burning around the electrodes; but from the start ECT showed some success in treating patients with severe depression. It is still in use in the 21st century for chronic depression that does not respond to other treatments, but nowadays patients are anesthetized and given a muscle relaxant first.

In 1935 Egas Moniz performed the world's first lobotomy in Portugal, disconnecting the frontal lobes from the parts of the brain that con-trolled emotion. The technique was designed to calm violent and uncontrollable patients, and it certainly did that, but it also left them lethargic, docile and lacking in emotion, and it had a high death rate of 25 percent. More than 40,000 lobotomies were performed in the United States and 17,000 in Britain, but the operation had fallen out

> *I got increasingly conservative about [lobotomy] because I don't think any of us were ever really happy about putting in a brain needle and stirring the works.*
> —**PSYCHIATRIST DR. JOHN PIPPARD, 1993**

of fashion by the 1960s. Playwright Tennessee Williams was an open critic after his sister Rose was permanently incapacitated by a lobotomy, and his play *Suddenly Last Summer* (1958) influenced public opinion.

PSYCHOPHARMACOLOGY

Australian physician John F.J. Cade had long been convinced that mental illness had a physiological cause. Others had tried to design mood-altering medicines and found the side effects proved worse than the original condition, but in 1949 Cade published a paper about lithium's ability to stabilize mood and prevent mania. When given to schizophrenics, it reduced hallucinations and made them less restless—but it did not seem effective when they were also experiencing depression. Further research produced the drug chlorpromazine, the first tranquilizer. By the 1960s diazepam (Valium) was widely prescribed to deal with everyday anxiety, and was referred to in the 1966 Rolling Stones song "Mother's Little Helper." It was followed in the 1980s by SSRIs (selective serotonin reuptake inhibitors), most famously Prozac.

The ability to treat mental illness with medication was a positive step forward, but it led to mass closures of mental health institutions, with disastrous effects for some patients, who struggled to look after themselves in society. Soon it was found that increasing percentages of the homeless and of prison inmates were experiencing some form of mental illness.

> *Freud was a hero. He descended to the Underworld and met there stark terrors. He carried with him his theory as a Medusa's head which turned these terrors to stone.*
> —R.D. LAING, *THE DIVIDED SELF*, 1960

Throughout the 20th century, the debate about the causes and treatment of mental illness continued. Scottish psychiatrist R.D. Laing argued that schizophrenia was caused by conflicted feelings in childhood, and he ran against the tide when he advocated that patients' experiences should be listened to and treated as valid. He was contradicted by American Franz Kallmann, who showed through twin studies that there is a hereditary element in psychiatric illness. By the end of the century, the consensus of opinion was that there can be a genetic predisposition that is triggered by traumatic life events, and treatment now tends to consist of a combination of drug therapy and talking cures.

Psychoanalysis has come a long way since Freud's insistence that childhood sexual guilt lay behind adult neuroses. There are now hundreds of different approaches to analysis, but Freud remains the one who popularized the talking cure and in the process became a household name.

Harold Gillies' Tubed Pedicle

LOCATION: Aldershot, England
DATE: 1917
FIELD: Surgery

Nose and ear reconstructions had been tried since ancient times with varying degrees of success, but the introduction of anesthesia and antisepsis in the 19th century meant that more sophisticated reconstructive surgery was possible. During the trench warfare of World War I, young men incurred appalling wounds to their faces and upper bodies, the parts that were most exposed to gun- and shellfire, and a pioneering New Zealand surgeon called Harold Gillies opened a specialty unit to try to restore some degree of normal appearance. Among his innovations was the tubed pedicle, an ingenious method of grafting skin onto damaged areas.

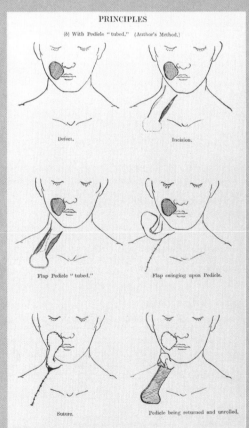

PRINCIPLES

(b) With Pedicle "tubed." (Author's Method.)

Defect. Incision.

Flap Pedicle "tubed." Flap swinging upon Pedicle.

Suture. Pedicle being returned and unrolled.

> *Within us all there is an overwhelming urge to change something ugly and useless into some other thing more beautiful and more functional.*
>
> —HAROLD GILLIES, SPEAKING AT THE FIRST INTERNATIONAL CONGRESS OF PLASTIC SURGERY IN STOCKHOLM, 1955

NOSE RECONSTRUCTION

The *Sushruta Samhita* of the first century BCE describes nose reconstruction after amputation (see page 21), and the Romans were able to reconstruct damaged ears around the same time. During the 15th century CE, Sicilian surgeon Antonio Branca devised a method of reconstructing a nose using a flap of skin from the arm, which involved strapping the patient's arm to his head for between 8 and 10 days while the blood supply was established before cutting the lower part of the graft free and making holes for nostrils. A century later this operation was described in *De Curtorum Chirurgia* (On the Surgery of the Maimed) by Gaspare Tagliacozzi, who used the method to reconstruct noses slashed off in duels, and also those lost due to syphilis.

During the 19th century, surgeons Félix Guyon of France, Jacques Reverdin of Switzerland and Carl Thiersch of Germany improved the technique of applying skin grafts; but the wounds remained open while the graft was being established, so they were prone to streptococcal and other kinds of bacterial infection for which, in those preantibiotic days, there was little that doctors could do.

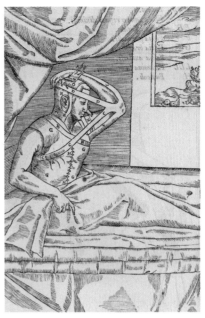

Reconstructing the nose with a skin graft from the arm was known as the "Italian method." The technique is shown here in an illustration by Gaspare Tagliacozzi, from 1597.

Syphilis

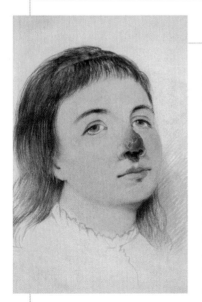

Syphilis is a sexually transmitted disease caused by the bacterium *Treponema pallidum*, which can be passed on congenitally. It was first recorded in Europe in 1495, and some epidemiologists think it was brought from the Americas by Christopher Columbus's crew. There were no effective cures until 1908, when Paul Ehrlich developed Salvarsan (see page 165); however, mercury was a common remedy, either inhaled, ingested, injected or rubbed on the skin, and many patients died of mercury poisoning. Symptoms included skin ulcers (as shown here), dementia, blindness and paralysis, but the most obvious sign was "saddle nose," where the bridge of the nose caved in and the flesh rotted away. This hole in the face led many people to wear artificial noses made of metal or leather, or seek surgeons willing to perform an early rhinoplasty.

THE ALDERSHOT PLASTIC SURGERY UNIT

When war was declared in 1914, Harold Gillies joined the Red Cross (see pages 124–27) and was sent to Belgium. On the way he encountered French surgeons Auguste Valadier, who was treating jaw wounds with skin grafts from elsewhere in the body, and Hippolyte Morestin, who let Gillies observe an operation for cancer of the face in which he used a roll of skin from beneath the patient's jaw to cover the wound.

Gillies was determined to work in this field of surgery, and in January 1916 he set up a unit at Aldershot military hospital in England and asked that all patients with jaw and facial injuries be sent to him. From the outset he determined that he did not want simply to heal wounds, but he also hoped to send the soldier back into the world with an appearance that was as good as, if not better than, before. He used sketches and wax models to plan his operations meticulously and took "before and after" photographs to document his work.

> *He invented plastic surgery. There was no plastic surgery before he came. Everything since then, no matter whose name be attached to it, was started by Gillies, perfected by him and handed on by him to lesser men, who have often claimed it as their own.*
>
> **—BRITISH PHYSICIAN SIR WILLIAM HENEAGE OGILVIE, 1962**

In October 1917 able seaman Willie Vicarage sustained appalling injuries in a cordite explosion on his ship. The skin was burned from his face; his eyelids and lower lip were turned inside out; and his nose became a twisted blob. Gillies cut a large flap of skin from the man's chest and pulled it up to cover his face, with apertures cut for the mouth and eyes, then brought thinner strips from the shoulders to anchor it. He found the skin had the tendency to curl inward, so he stitched the edges of the flaps together to create a tube of living tissue. This had the benefits of increasing the flow of blood to the graft while sealing off raw tissue to prevent infection. It was also less liable to degeneration than unsewn grafts. The tubed pedicle was born, and it showed such dramatic results that patients all over Gillies' wards were soon sprouting these strange-looking tubes. Once the graft had taken, they were cut off, having performed their role.

Gillies' innovations did not stop there. He invented a technique to restore lost

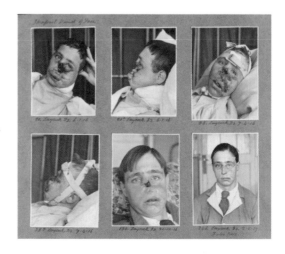

Soldiers with shrapnel wounds, 1916–18. Facial injuries were common in World War I as the head was more exposed than the rest of the body in trench warfare. (Image courtesy of Army Medical Services Museum)

eyelids; he reconstructed an entire nose using a section of cartilage from the patient's ribs; he designed an intranasal skin graft for people with leprosy; and he also devised new methods for reattaching severed limbs. During the war, he performed more than 11,000 operations on more than 5,000 men, both at Aldershot and later at a special plastic surgery hospital in Sidcup, Kent.

THE GUINEA PIGS' CLUB

In 1932 Gillies hired a distant cousin, Archibald McIndoe, to work with him, and just before the start of World War II McIndoe became consultant surgeon to the Royal Air Force. During the Battle of Britain, 4,000 young pilots received terrible facial burns from fuel that ignited after their planes were shot down. Some of them were so badly disfigured that they needed up to 30 operations to restore their features, and McIndoe recognized that social reintegration would be an important part of their recovery. He urged local people in the East Grinstead area to invite the pilots for tea and reassure them that their appearance was acceptable in society. Aware that the operations being performed on them were groundbreaking, patients formed what they called The Guinea Pigs' Club, with Archibald McIndoe as its lifelong president.

McIndoe developed the tubular graft into what was known as the walking-stick or waltzing graft, which was periodically detached and anchored closer to the target site. He also recognized that saline can help wound healing after observing the difference in recovery times between pilots shot down over land and at sea.

After the war, both McIndoe and Gillies moved into private practice. McIndoe was known for his cosmetic work on reshaping the nose, whereas Gillies performed a range of procedures, including one of the first gender reassignment operations, when he performed a phalloplasty in 1946 on Laurence Michael Dillon, who had been assigned female at birth.

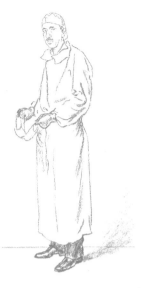

Harold Gillies was a keen painter in his spare time and exhibited his work in London in 1948. This aesthetic talent helped in his surgical reconstruction of damaged faces.

Cosmetic Surgery

A distinction is drawn between reconstructive surgery—which corrects impairments caused by burns, traumatic injuries, congenital abnormalities (such as cleft palate), infections or diseases, cancer or tumors—and cosmetic surgery, which is optional and undertaken to improve appearance or reverse the signs of aging. After World War II, a range of factors led to a demand for cosmetic surgery: the eugenics movement in the United States, the proliferation of beauty contests and the popularity of movies and TV programs with seemingly perfect stars. The top five cosmetic procedures are now breast augmentation, liposuction, nose reshaping, eyelid surgery and tummy tucks.

Spanish Flu Mask

LOCATION:	Worldwide
DATE:	1918–19
FIELD:	Epidemiology

In March 1918 a soldier reported to the hospital in Fort Riley, Kansas, with a cough and fever; within a week there were 500 men with the same symptoms and just over a year later, the influenza outbreak had killed somewhere between 25 and 50 million people worldwide. No one knew what was causing it and rumors spread that the Germans were using a biological weapon of warfare—but their troops were affected just as much as the Allies'. At first the epidemic was not widely reported except in Spain, which was not fighting in the war, hence the name "Spanish flu." There were no effective treatments, but people wore gauze masks in an attempt to prevent the spread of the terrifying disease.

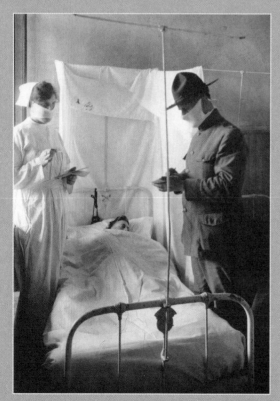

If the epidemic continues its mathematical rate of acceleration, civilization could easily disappear from the face of the earth within a few weeks.
—VICTOR VAUGHAN, SURGEON GENERAL OF THE U.S. ARMY, OCTOBER 1918

FROM KANSAS TO THE WORLD'S REMOTEST SPOTS

At first no one paid much attention to the flu that appeared to originate in Fort Riley, Kansas, in March 1918. It seemed a mild strain, and there were more important matters occupying the public attention, because the United States had entered World War I the year before and thousands of troopships were crossing the Atlantic to take soldiers to the Western Front. By April cases were appearing in France, where some thought it could be a side effect of the mustard gas that had been used as a weapon, or a result of the smoke and fumes of war. The Germans were equally affected, with General von Ludendorff blaming the flu for halting a planned German advance in July 1918.

In September, a new strain of flu emerged in Boston, Massachusetts. This one caused piercing headaches, a severe cough and a high fever, and within days or even hours, patients' faces turned blue from cyanosis. They were succumbing to a form of bacterial pneumonia leading to acute respiratory distress syndrome. Their lungs filled with fluid and they had uncontrollable nosebleeds, with blood-tinged sputum foaming from their mouth and nose. The mortality rate was 10 to 20 percent, a massive increase on the 0.1 percent rate for previous flu outbreaks. And unlike other flu viruses, which mostly killed children and the elderly, this one was also affecting healthy people in their prime, between 20 and 40 years old.

The epidemic spread rapidly along shipping lines and following troop movements. In Fiji, 14 percent of the population died within 2 weeks of its arrival; it claimed 22 percent of Western Samoans. The epidemic subsided in November 1918, when the Armistice to end the war was signed, but street celebrations after the declaration of peace may have triggered a resurgence that lasted from December 1918 to May 1919. By then as many as one third of the world's population had caught it and between 3 and 5 percent had perished—up to three times as many as those who died in the war.

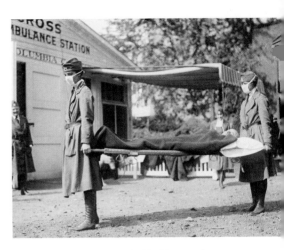

Masked Red Cross workers carry an influenza patient in Washington, D.C. There were no vaccines or drugs to combat the virus; the only treatment offered was Epsom salts.

Gauze Masks

Doctors in the early 20th century had no cures for influenza, although Epsom salts were commonly recommended. Public gatherings were banned at the height of the epidemic, with schools, stores and businesses closed, and gauze face masks were worn outdoors to try to protect the wearer. Flu virus is spread by droplets in the coughs or sneezes of those with the infection, which can persist on surfaces for up to 24 hours. Someone touching that surface and then touching their own mouth, nose or eyes can be infected. Masks provided protection from airborne droplets, but these could linger on the gauze and be transferred onto the hands as the wearer took them off in what they thought was the safety of their own home, thus doing more harm than good.

CAUSES AND CURES

There was a major breakthrough in understanding influenza in 1933 when Christopher Andrewes and Wilson Smith at the National Institute for Medical Research in London inoculated ferrets with material taken from the back of Andrewes' throat while he was sick with flu. A few days later the ferrets were sneezing and feverish. One of the ferrets sneezed in the face of a researcher and he came down with flu, thus proving that the virus was capable of leaping between species.

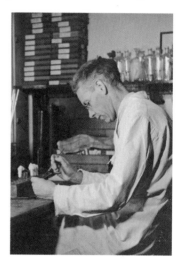

Left: Electron micrograph of the 1918 flu virus that killed more people than the Black Death had at its height in 1347–51 (see pages 56–61). Below: Christopher Andrewes in the London laboratory where he helped to identify the virus that causes influenza type A.

Ten years later, in 1943, the electron microscope enabled scientists to see the flu virus for the first time, and an understanding was reached of how the virus needs a living host to enable it to reproduce.

Flu appears every winter, but humans build up immunity to normal strains. However, epidemics occur when a virus emerges that has mutated into a new strain, a process known as "antigenic drift." The H1N1 strain that caused the Spanish flu outbreak may have mutated when a soldier in a military camp was exposed to avian flu from chickens while he also had human flu, allowing the viruses to mix.

In 1997, pathologist Johan Hultin collected a sample of Spanish flu virus from a mass grave in the tiny Alaskan town of Brevig, where the victim, whom he named "Lucy," was preserved in the permafrost. He was able to examine the RNA

The Discovery of Viruses

In 1884, French microbiologist Charles Chamberland developed a filter with pores that did not allow bacteria to pass through. In the following decade, researchers found that sap from an infected tobacco plant remained infectious when passed through this filter. Chamberland argued that the infectious agent must still be there, and named it a virus. In 1931, U.S. pathologist Ernest William Goodpasture was able to grow the influenza virus in chickens' eggs; then in 1949 the polio virus was grown (see pages 160–63). During the 1950s a number of new viruses were isolated for the first time, including the rhinoviruses that cause the common cold. In 1964 British researchers Michael Epstein and Yvonne Barr published a paper showing how the Epstein–Barr virus caused cancer—the first virus known to do so. Since then, many new viruses have been discovered, including HIV (see pages 202–205) and Ebola (see pages 214–17).

(ribonucleic acid, a molecule like DNA that conveys genetic information) and identify three genes that weakened the bronchial tubes and the lungs, clearing the way for bacterial pneumonia to set in. He also showed how the virus overstimulated the immune system, causing a cytokine storm (see page 216), and that's why those with the healthiest immune systems were most likely to perish.

BIRD FLU SCARES

In May 1957 a pandemic that came to be known as Asian flu was first reported in Hong Kong (although it is thought to have started in mainland China) and spread around the world on shipping routes. This H2N2 virus primarily affected children, who had no immunity to previous flu strains, and the global death toll was two million, despite the production of an effective vaccine. In July 1968 there was another H2N2 outbreak in Hong Kong, but the death toll was lower at 750,000, probably because some had immunity from the Asian flu outbreak 11 years earlier.

An H5N1 virus spread through chickens and ducks in 1987 and a decade later the first instance was recorded of its infecting a human; 18 human cases were noted in Hong Kong, of whom six died. There was a widespread cull of domestic birds amid fears of an epidemic, but as of 2012 only 359 humans had died of H5N1. In 2013 a deadly H7N9 virus appeared in China, but it seems that prompt action to close markets selling wild birds prevented it from turning into a global pandemic.

A Chinese bird market is inspected for signs of avian flu in 2014. Such markets have proved a breeding ground for new strains of flu because humans and animals are in close proximity.

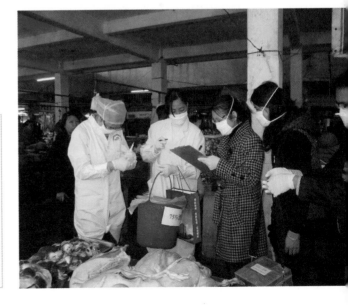

The clock keeps ticking. Every time this virus replicates, it makes mistakes ... Sooner or later it will make the mistakes that will allow it to go human to human.
—VIROLOGIST ROBERT WEBSTER ON BIRD FLU, *AMERICAN SCIENTIST*, 2003

Lilly's Insulin Syringe

LOCATION: Toronto, Canada
DATE: 1923
FIELD: Endocrinology

Doctors in ancient times recognized the symptoms of diabetes—an Indian physician noted in 1500 BCE that the sweetness of his patient's urine attracted ants—but for the next 35 centuries it was more often than not a death sentence. No one had any idea what caused the disease until the 19th century, when it was found to be linked with secretions from the pancreas. In 1921 Frederick Banting and Charles Best managed to keep a severely diabetic dog alive by injecting it with canine insulin, and the race was on to find a source from which large quantities of insulin suitable for use in humans could be produced. Their work would save millions of lives.

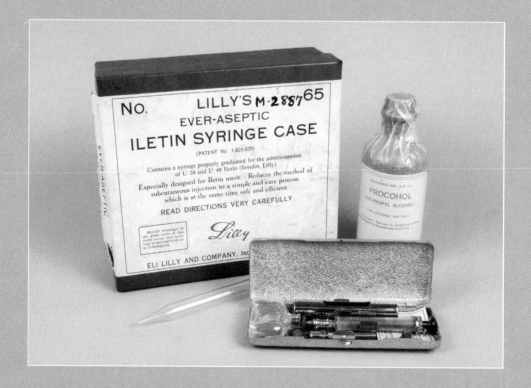

FROM OIL OF ROSES TO INSULIN

The physician Areteus of Cappadocia (ca. first or second century CE) recommended oil of roses, dates, raw quinces and gruel for patients who presented with the symptoms of diabetes: frequent urination, excessive thirst, unusual tiredness, blurred vision and genital itching, combined with sweet-tasting urine. One 17th-century remedy included "gelly of viper's flesh, broken red coral, sweet almonds, and fresh flowers of blind nettles." However, for most people with type 1 diabetes before the 20th century, the outlook was bleak. The cells in the pancreas that produce insulin were missing or degenerated, and as a result the sugar in their blood could not be taken up by the muscles or adipose tissue. Hyperglycemia (excess of sugar in the bloodstream) eventually caused them to become drowsy or fall into a coma, and many died a painful, wasting death, gasping for air as they tried to expel carbon dioxide from their lungs.

No one had yet discovered the role of hormones in the body, but in 1889 Oskar Minkowski and Joseph von Mering found that dogs developed sweet-smelling urine and other diabetes symptoms after the removal of their pancreas. Two decades earlier, German pathologist Paul Langerhans had identified clusters of cells in the pancreas, which were later named the islets of Langerhans. In 1902, following the work of Bayliss and Starling on the influence of hormones, it was discovered that these islets were responsible for producing a substance called insulin, and that lack of insulin was the cause of diabetes symptoms.

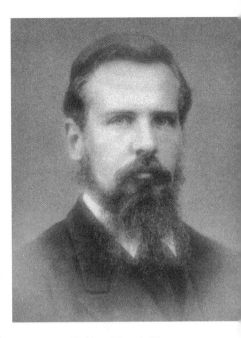

Working with a primitive light microscope, Paul Langherans made incredibly detailed pictures of a number of cells, including the insulin-secreting cells in the pancreas that are named after him.

The Many Roles of Hormones

In 1893 British physiologists George Oliver and Edward Schafer injected a dog with an extract from an adrenal gland, and noted that its blood pressure went sky-high. In 1902 William Bayliss and Henry Starling noted that the duodenum secreted a substance that traveled through the blood to stimulate the pancreas to produce "pancreatic juice." The term "hormone" was coined for these chemical messengers, from a Greek word meaning "to excite or arouse." Before World War I, Dr. Harvey Cushing of Baltimore, Maryland, had discovered the role of the pituitary gland in the control of the endocrine system. And in 1923 Edward Doisy and Edgar Allen in St. Louis, Missouri, extracted female sex hormones and created the first pregnancy test by injecting a woman's urine into lab rats or mice and watching to see if they went into heat.

BANTING AND BEST

In 1921 Canadian physician Frederick Banting was determined to find a way for diabetics to replace the insulin their bodies were not producing. Working in the University of Toronto laboratory of Professor John Macleod, with his lab assistant Charles Best, Banting managed to extract insulin from a dog's islets of Langerhans. They injected it into a diabetic dog that was close to death and within a few hours the dog was wagging its tail and barking. A local slaughterhouse supplied them with insulin from cattle and they found that it worked on diabetic dogs; they then did the first human trial on themselves. In January 1922 Banting injected a 14-year-old boy who was dying of diabetes; his blood sugar fell to normal levels immediately, and within weeks he was home from the hospital. Biochemist James Collip helped them to purify insulin extract, and they demonstrated that daily injections would help to control diabetes.

Banting and Best: When the Nobel Prize for Medicine was awarded to Banting and Macleod in 1923, Banting split his prize money with Best.

Insulin production at Eli Lilly and Company in the 1930s. Back then, insulin was obtained from the pancreases of animals, particularly cattle and pigs.

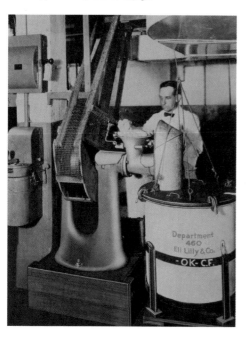

Diet and Diabetes

It was long recognized that diet could influence diabetes; about 1000 BCE it was recommended that diabetics eat a diet of wheat grains, grapes, honey and berries. At the beginning of the 20th century, Dr. Frederick Allen of New Jersey advised patients to eat just 450 calories a day, which pro- longed life but made them very weak. In 1927, Dr. Elliott Joslin of Boston recommend- ed a diet of 2 percent carbohydrates, 20 percent protein and 75 percent fat, believing that diabetics could not tolerate carbs. In the 1970s, when fat was blamed for an increase in cardiovascular disease, the recommendation was that it should not account for more than 30 percent of calorie intake—but this led to the consumption of more carbohydrates, which led to increased obesity. Now the advice is to have a healthy, balanced diet, that is low in salt, sugar and saturated fat.

Eli Lilly and Company began to manufacture insulin in 1923, marketing it under the brand name Iletin. It had to be injected, since it breaks down in the digestive system; so as well as bottles of insulin, Eli Lilly sold a kit called the Ever-Antiseptic Iletin Syringe Case, which contained a syringe, spare needles, a glass pipette, cotton balls, a small bottle with a rubber cap in which to carry the insulin and some isopropyl alcohol to sterilize the syringe. Banting and Best had not given them an exclusive licence to manufacture insulin, but Iletin was still one of the best-selling products in the company's history, allowing diabetics to treat themselves at home.

The needles were enormous, and they came with little pumice stones so that you could sharpen them. They often became dull and developed barbs on the end. And in order to sterilize them they had to be boiled for 20 minutes.
—DR. NANCY BOHANNON, DIABETES HEALTH BOARD, DESCRIBING EARLY INSULIN SYRINGES

IMPROVING THE LIVES OF DIABETICS

In 1935, Roger Hinsworth discovered that there were two types of diabetes— insulin-insensitive (type 1) and insulin-sensitive (type 2)— and in the 1950s oral drugs called sulfonylureas were introduced to help manage blood sugar levels for those with type 2. Further medicines have been developed since then, but type 2 cases now account for 90 percent of all diabetes in the developed world as a consequence of high levels of obesity.

Before the 1950s, blood sugar levels were tested using a substance called Benedict's solution, which had to be mixed with urine and heated over boiling water, but in 1953 the first test strips for urine were introduced. In 1969 a blood glucose meter was developed that would be invaluable in hospital emergency departments for distinguishing between those who were in a diabetic coma and those who had drunk themselves unconscious. And in 1976 the first insulin pumps appeared, which deliver small, regular amounts of insulin through a catheter without the need for injections. In 1978 a biotechnology company called Genentech developed the first synthetic insulin from genetically altered bacteria, and today's nanotechnologists (see page 201) are testing a "smart delivery" system of measuring glucose and delivering insulin at molecular level in the bloodstream.

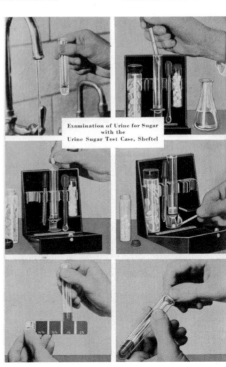

A case for testing the amount of sugar in urine, produced by Eli Lilly in 1942. It was a complicated business that required diabetics to keep rows of test tubes on their bathroom windowsill.

Examination of Urine for Sugar with the Urine Sugar Test Case, Sheftel

The Iron Lung

LOCATION:	Boston, Massachusetts
DATE:	1928
FIELD:	Biomedical engineering, life support

No drugs have the slightest influence upon acute myelitis. The child should be put to bed and the affected limb or limbs wrapped in cotton.
—CANADIAN PHYSICIAN
WILLIAM OSLER, 1892

It was every parent's nightmare: A previously healthy child complained of a stiff neck and back, then felt a little feverish, and within hours might be totally paralyzed. Poliomyelitis causes irreversible paralysis in one of every 200 cases, and of those with paralytic polio, 2 to 5 percent of children and 15 to 30 percent of adults die. There were epidemics of polio in the United States every summer throughout the late 19th century and the first half of the 20th, and no one could find a cure; but two Boston engineers created a machine called the iron lung, which could keep victims alive by taking over their breathing for them.

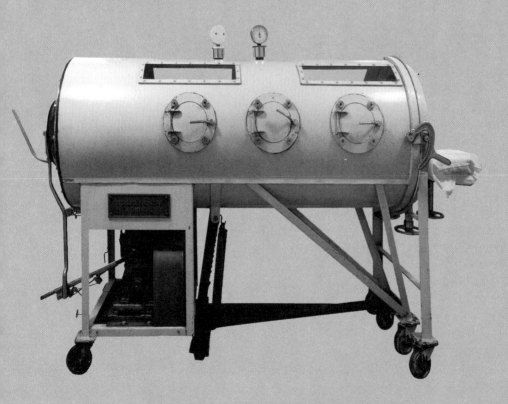

ARTIFICIAL RESPIRATION

An Egyptian stele (carved stone slab) of 1403–1365 BCE shows a priest with a club foot supporting himself on a walking stick, an indication that he might have had polio as a child. The disease became more prevalent after the growth of cities in the 19th and early 20th centuries, with 27,000 new cases reported in the United States in 1916, and 6,000 polio-related deaths in that year alone.

The poliomyelitis virus is transmitted through ingested feces and swimming pools were a common place to pick it up, but this was not realized until 1940. Although most patients fight it off, in an unlucky few with "paralytic polio" it enters the nervous system, destroying the motor neurons in the spinal cord responsible for the muscles of the trunk, limbs and chest. It most commonly affects children, but President Franklin D. Roosevelt caught it at the age of 39 and was left paralyzed from the waist down.

There had been attempts to produce artificial respirators from the 17th century, when they were used to try to save victims of drowning. Early prototypes were like bellows that forced air into the lungs, but there was no control over the force and too powerful a blast could damage internal organs. In 1889 Dr. O.W. Doe developed an infant respirator in which a child's mouth was pressed

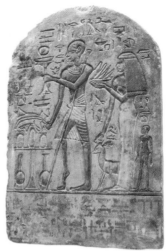

This stele dating from 1403–1365 BCE showing a priest named Rema with an emaciated leg, leaning on a staff, is the main evidence that polio existed in ancient Egypt.

Haldane's Coffin

Scottish physiologist John Haldane spent his career exploring the effect of gases on the human body, and to that end he carried out a series of experiments in which he and a colleague were locked in a sealed box (known as Haldane's coffin), breathing and rebreathing the air and noting the effects. He investigated several mine disasters and found that carbon monoxide poisoning was asphyxiating miners. He recommended they take white mice or canaries underground because these would succumb first and provide an early warning. In 1907 Haldane invented a decompression chamber for divers, and when poison gas was used during World War I, he invented the gas mask.

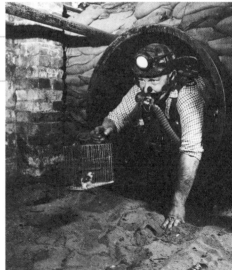

A Welsh miner uses a canary to test for methane and carbon dioxide. Canaries swayed on their perches when even small amounts were present in the atmosphere.

against a diaphragm and its body encased in a wooden box, while an operator blew into a pipe 20 or 30 times a minute to force the chest to compress. In 1928 Philip Drinker and Louis Agassiz Shaw of Harvard University took this principle several stages further by developing a respirator powered by an electric motor, with pumps that sucked air in and out of a vacuum-sealed cylinder. They originally designed it to treat victims of coal gas poisoning but it was almost immediately adopted to save the lives of those with paralytic polio.

THE IRON LUNG

Being pushed into Drinker and Shaw's original iron lung while struggling for breath was intimidating for young polio victims, so in 1931 John Emerson produced a version with a few modifications. This had a bed, known as the "cookie tray," on which patients could be slid in and out of the cylinder, and there were portal windows in the side through which nurses could remove bedpans, adjust sheets and scratch a patient's itches. A mirror was positioned so that the immobilized patient could see what was going on in the room. Most patients spent 1 to 2 weeks in an iron lung until they were able to breathe independently again, but some stayed in it for the rest of their lives. At the height of the outbreaks of the 1940s and 1950s, rows of iron lungs filled hospital wards.

Scientists were trying to find a vaccine to protect against polio, and after trials in 1935 in which six children died, President Roosevelt established a National Foundation for Infant Paralysis (NFIP) and put huge funding behind it. By the late 1940s the fact that the virus was

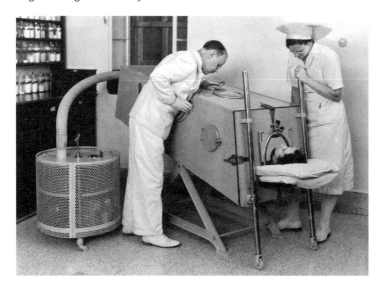

A polio patient in an iron lung at a hospital in Palestine, 1940. At the time, each machine cost $1,500, about the same as an average family home in the United States.

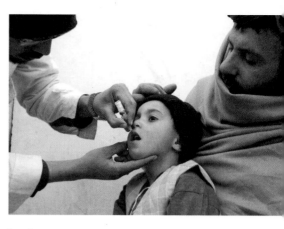

A child in Pakistan is given the polio vaccine as part of the ongoing eradication campaign. In October 2015 the country had 38 reported cases, the highest worldwide.

transmitted by feces had been discovered, and in 1951 researchers found that there were three separate strains. In 1955 Jonas Salk at Pittsburgh University developed an inactivated virus that protected the nervous system; but it did not eradicate the virus from the digestive system, so polio could still spread. His vaccine also required a course of injections, but it was the system adopted in the United States at the time.

In Cincinnati, Ohio, Albert Sabin developed a live attenuated vaccine that was taken orally. The NFIP would not support his live trials in the United States, but between 1957 and 1959 he conducted trials in the USSR, Eastern Europe, Mexico and elsewhere. The results were positive. His vaccine eradicated all three types of polio in one oral dose, which could be taken in a sugar cube or a spoonful of sugar syrup. From 1962 it became the most widely used polio vaccine.

THE FIGHT TO ERADICATE POLIO

In 1988 the World Health Organization (see pages 176–7) started a Global Polio Eradication Initiative; since then, more than 2.5 billion children have been inoculated and the number of new cases has decreased by more than 99 percent. Polio is still endemic in Pakistan and Afghanistan, and there are signs that it may be recurring in Syria, since it is difficult to inoculate children in war-torn countries.

In 1959 there were 1,200 people in iron lungs in U.S. hospitals, but by 2014 there were only 10 remaining. Artificial respiration is mostly done by ventilators now, inserted through the mouth or via a tracheotomy tube.

Life Support

In the 21st century, modern hospital equipment can take over many of the functions of human organs and systems. A ventilator or respirator will pump air into the lungs when patients are unable to breathe independently. If the heart stops, doctors try cardiopulmonary resuscitation, defibrillation or medication to start it again, and a heart-lung bypass machine (see pages 170–71) can take over for up to 10 hours during cardiac surgery. Dialysis machines can perform the function of the kidneys (see pages 174–75), and feeding tubes can supply all the nutrients and liquids a patient needs. Life support is usually a stopgap solution to support a patient during recovery from an underlying problem, but it can be used long-term in certain circumstances.

Alexander Fleming's Petri Dish

LOCATION:	London, England
DATE:	1928
FIELD:	Bacteriology, immunology

Alexander Fleming was researching influenza when he accidentally left some staphylococcus bacteria uncovered in a Petri dish while on a 3-week vacation. When he returned, he saw that spores of airborne mold had landed on the dish and appeared to have killed the bacteria in their vicinity. He did not believe this observation would have practical applications but published a paper about it anyway. Twelve years later his discovery was taken up by some Australian researchers and the modern antibiotic era began. Penicillin was hailed as the new wonder drug— between 1942 and 1975 global life expectancy shot up by 8 years when cures were found for diseases, such as tuberculosis, that had previously been major killers.

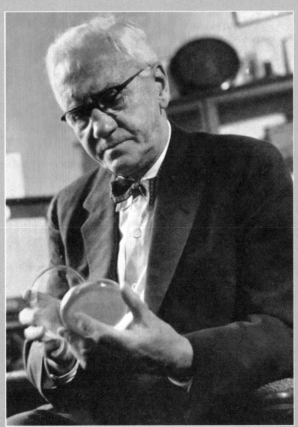

One sometimes finds what one is not looking for
—ALEXANDER FLEMING,
NOBEL PRIZE LECTURE, 1945

THE APPLICATIONS OF MOLD

The ancient Greeks, Romans and Indians had used plant and bread molds to treat infection based not on an understanding of how they worked but simply on folklore about their efficacy. The scientists of the late 19th century were edging toward an understanding of bacteria: Louis Pasteur (see pages 114–19) noticed that some bacteria are antagonistic to other bacteria and speculated that this might be harnessed for therapeutic purposes, whereas Joseph Lister (see pages 128–31) experimented with the antibacterial action of *Penicillium glaucum*, the mold found on blue cheeses. In 1897 Ernest Duchesne healed some guinea pigs with typhoid using *P. glaucum*, but his work received little attention.

German physician Paul Ehrlich noticed that chemical dyes were taken up by some bacteria and not others, and concluded that it should be possible to kill bacteria selectively without harming surrounding cells. This led to the production in 1909 of the antibacterial drug Salvarsan, which Ehrlich called "chemotherapy." It was the first effective treatment for syphilis but had some nasty side effects, so it was not universally hailed as a breakthrough.

In 1928 Fleming did not appreciate the importance of his accidental discovery of the way *P. notatum* mold (now called *P. chrysogenum*) killed staphylococcus bacteria in a Petri dish. When exploring the biological properties of the mold juice, he found that an active substance in it was still effective when diluted 800 times. He called this ingredient "penicillin" but did not think it would be possible to extract and produce it in large enough quantities for widespread use, so he simply published a paper about it in the *British Journal of Experimental Pathology* and went back to his other work.

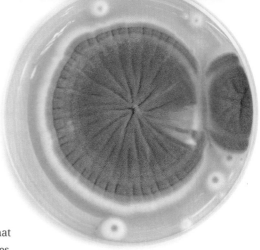

There are more than 300 varieties of *Penicillium* fungi. They cause foods to spoil and mold to grow in damp buildings, as well as having medical uses.

Leading Causes of Mortality

In 1900 the top three causes of mortality in the United States were pneumonia/influenza, tuberculosis and diarrheal diseases, with heart disease fourth, stroke fifth and cancer eighth. In 1920 pneumonia/influenza was still the number one killer but heart disease had risen to second, with tuberculosis third, diarrhea eighth and puerperal infections tenth. By 1950, when antibiotics were available, heart disease was the number one killer, cancer second and pneumonia and tuberculosis had dropped to sixth and seventh, respectively. By 1954 tuberculosis had left the top 10 entirely, as had puerperal fever. Today, the top three killers are heart disease, cancer and chronic respiratory diseases.

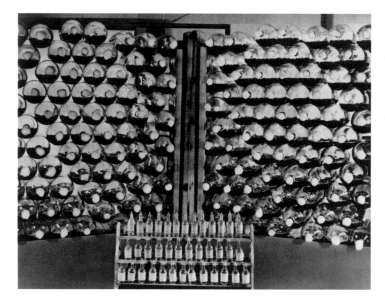

Mass production of penicillin during World War II. By 1945, a strain had been developed that was 10 times more potent than the best strain available in 1939.

FROM LAB TO BATTLEFIELD

During the 1930s, while looking for antibacterial substances, Australian scientists Howard Florey and Ernst Chain came across Fleming's paper. They grew *Penicillium notatum* in their lab and in 1940 tested it on mice with streptococcus infections; those given the medicine survived whereas the rest died. Florey and Chain went to the United States for help with mass production of penicillin, and the U.S. government gave financial backing after the medicine was successfully used to treat victims of a devastating 1942 fire in a Boston nightclub. Normally, skin grafts carried a high risk of infection (see pages 148–51), but penicillin treatment helped those burns victims to survive. The race was on to produce enough of the "wonder drug" to help Allied soldiers fighting in World War II, and by D-Day in June 1944, there was enough for every Allied serviceman. The secret was kept from the Germans, Japanese and Italians until after the war, and as a result they had many more cases of limb amputation from wound infection.

> *The first rule of antibiotics is try not to use them, and the second rule is try not to use too many of them.*
> —P.L. MARINO, "ANTIMICROBIAL THERAPY,"
> IN *THE ICU BOOK*, 2007

Biochemists turned their attention to creating new antibiotics to treat a range of different bacterial infections. Some, such as penicillin, metronizadole and cotrimoxazole, were bacteridical: they killed bacteria by interfering with their cell formation. Others, such as the tetracyclines and sulfonamides, were bacteriostatic, meaning that they stopped bacteria from multiplying. Suddenly there were cures for tuberculosis, whooping cough, gonorrhea, pneumonia, urinary tract infections, puerperal fever, scarlet fever, bacterial meningitis and a range of diarrheal diseases that would previously have been fatal. In the preantibiotic days, even the most minor operations carried a risk of postoperative infection, but after 1945 surgeons could attempt more complex surgery than they would ever have tried before. It seemed truly miraculous.

ANTIBIOTIC RESISTANCE

Back in 1945, Fleming had warned that too small a dose of antibiotics might fail to completely clear an infection, leading to microbes developing resistance to the drugs. In fact, there would be positive selection of resistant bacteria because they were the ones that survived. His advice was not heeded, and instead penicillin was soon freely available to the public in all kinds of over-the-counter forms: as salves, creams, ointments, lozenges and tablets. In 1955 it would become available only with a prescription in the United States, but already penicillin-resistant staphylococci had emerged. In 1959 a synthetic penicillin called methicillin was created, but methicillin-resistant *Staphylococcus aureus* (MRSA) emerged 2 years later. The problem was overprescription of antibiotics for illnesses they could not treat, such as influenza and colds, and in some countries antibiotics were used as prophylactics (to prevent infection), giving resistant microbes a chance to develop.

In the 21st century, antibiotic-resistant infections are increasingly emerging and few new antibiotics are being developed. Every year there are half a million cases of antibiotic-resistant tuberculosis, and the fear is that unless new medicines are developed we could return to the early days of the 20th century when bacterial infections meant a death sentence, or at the very least amputation of the affected body part.

Superbugs

Drug-resistant superbugs often appear in hospitals, where both the bacteria and the medicines used to fight them are found in close proximity. MRSA is a bacterium that is commonly carried on the skin, where it causes minor infections, but if it gets into the bloodstream through an open wound or a catheter, it can be extremely difficult to treat, with a mortality rate of between 20 and 35 percent. *Clostridium difficile*, which causes intestinal infections, kills 14,000 people a year, and patients are more likely to catch it after a course of antibiotics has damaged the balance of healthy intestinal bacteria. Carbapenem-resistant Enterobacteriaceae (a large family of bacteria, some harmful and some not) cause infections in the bloodstream and kill 600 annually; and *Neisseria gonorrheae*, which causes gonorrhea, has strains that are currently resistant to all medication.

Electron micrograph of methicillin-resistant Staphylococcus aureus (MRSA) being ingested by a white blood cell.

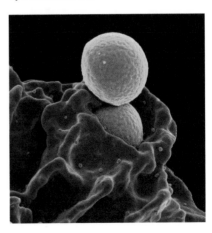

Bryukhonenko's Autojektor

LOCATION: Moscow, USSR
DATE: 1928
FIELD: Surgery, physiology

In the first half of the 20th century, physiologists turned their attention to ways of keeping organs alive and supplied with oxygenated blood when the body was no longer capable of doing so. In the United States a major focus of research was developing a heart-lung machine that could take over when the heart was temporarily stopped to allow open-heart surgery. In Russia the challenge was even more dramatic: Could they bring organs back to life using the autojektor machine invented by Sergei Bryukhonenko? Today, these experiments might seem unethical, but they opened up some interesting questions—including what exactly is meant by the term "death."

> *Vague reports have been reaching the U.S. that Russian scientists have revivified corpses.*
> —*TIME* MAGAZINE, 1929

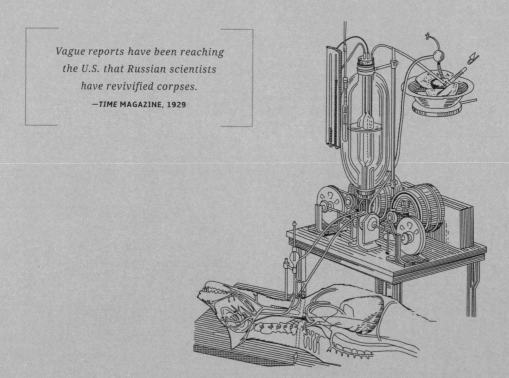

BACK FROM THE DEAD

During the 1880s British physiologist Frank Spiller Locke developed a saline solution that could keep excised hearts beating in the physiology lab. This was useful for research purposes but he never imagined the uses to which it would later be put. In 1902 Alexei Kulyabko, working in St. Petersburg, Russia, used Locke's solution to restart a rabbit's heart that had stopped beating 44 hours earlier, and the following year he did the same with the heart of a baby who had died of pneumonia. Between 1910 and 1913, Fyodor Andreyev took this a step further when he resuscitated a dog by injecting it with saline and adrenaline, then applying electric shocks to the heart.

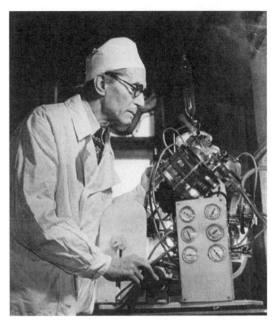

Sergei Bryukhonenko with his autojektor, one of the earliest heart-lung machines. It used the lungs of a donor animal to oxygenate the blood, and two pumps to circulate it through the system and back into the subject.

None of these creatures stayed "alive" for long, but the possibilities intrigued the Moscow scientist Sergei Bryukhonenko. He designed a machine that would replenish an animal's blood by first pumping it out, warming and oxygenating it in a glass jar, then pumping it back in. In 1928, at the Third Congress of Physiologists in Moscow, Bryukhonenko demonstrated his autojektor being used on the severed head of a dog. As the reoxygenated blood circulated, the head began to react to external stimuli, notably blinking when a bright light was shone into its eye.

The Definition of Death

The 1768 edition of *Encyclopedia Britannica* defined death as the separation of soul and body, and this belief is reflected in the cave paintings and funeral rituals of many civilizations. Up to the mid-20th century, physicians declared a person dead if the heart was no longer beating and air did not flow in and out of the lungs, and some pinched the skin to confirm that there was no pain response. The problem was that a growing number of patients could be revived from such a state with mouth-to-mouth respiration and chest compressions. Technological advances in monitoring made it possible to propose a lack of electrical activity in the brain as a definition of death—but which part of the brain? The term "information-theoretic death" was coined to mean the destruction of the brain to such an extent that recovery of cerebral function would be impossible. The debate continues as technology advances.

Taking these experiments to a logical conclusion, in 1929 Kulyabko and Andreyev attempted to "reanimate" a man who had passed away during surgery the previous day. After they had pumped his blood with Locke's solution and adrenaline, his heart heaved in his chest and a choking sound came from his throat. He was kept "alive" in this way for 20 minutes. In 1934 Sergei Spasokukotsky revived a man who had committed suicide 3 hours earlier. Using the autojektor he restored a heartbeat and heard sounds in the throat, but when the man's eyelids opened the shocked scientist quickly switched off the machine to let him "die" again.

> *Rarely, if ever, has one single research effort expanded so much the capacity of surgeons to be of help to the congenitally malformed and to those disabled by acquired lesions.*
> —**HARRIS B. SHUMACKER**, *JOHN HEYSHAM GIBBON JR., 1903–1973 (1982)*

HEART-LUNG MACHINES

German scientist Maximilian von Frey had constructed an early prototype heart-lung machine back in 1885, but it was not feasible to use it in practice until the discovery in 1916 that heparin could be used to prevent blood coagulation—and even then it was not particularly successful. In October 1930, American surgeon John Heysham Gibbon Jr. was part of a team that operated to remove a massive pulmonary embolism from a female patient. When she subsequently died, he became determined to devise an effective heart-lung machine and devoted the next 23 years of his life to this research.

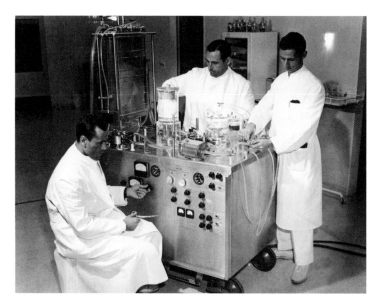

A heart-lung machine in 1958. Throughout the 1950s and 1960s, heart surgery became more successful with advances in diagnosis, anti-coagulation methods and postoperative care, as well as the new machines.

Gibbon's first design, a cylinder in which oxygen was blown onto a thin film of blood, could not work fast enough. It was only when he covered the inside of the cylinder with wire mesh to create turbulence and increase the surface area that enough blood was oxygenated per minute to support life. On May 6, 1953, he used his machine for 26 minutes while closing a septal defect in the heart of an 18-year-old woman. The operation was a complete success and she was discharged 13 days later.

CARDIAC SURGERY

Before John Gibbon's breakthrough, few heart operations were attempted. Some 19th-century surgeons had operated on the pericardium surrounding the heart, but in 1896, when Dr. Ludwig Rehn of Frankfurt, Germany, repaired damage to the right ventricle caused by a stab wound, it was the first successful heart operation. In 1925, British surgeon Henry Souttar operated on a patient with mitral stenosis (a narrowing of the mitral valve), and in 1947 another British doctor, Thomas Holmes Sellors, operated on a patient with pulmonary stenosis, which obstructed the blood flow from the right ventricle to the pulmonary artery. During the 1940s and 1950s a team of surgeons at Johns Hopkins University in Baltimore, Maryland, developed a successful operation to treat blue babies born with congenital heart malforma-tions, by joining the subclavian artery to the pulmonary artery. That was as far as surgeons could go without stopping the heart from beating and thus stopping the circulation of oxygenated blood to the brain and other organs.

After the development of successful heart-lung machines, it became possible to treat all kinds of complex heart defects, cardiac valve disorders, atherosclerotic obstructions of the coronary artery and aneurisms of the thoracic aorta. The groundwork was laid that would enable Christiaan Barnard to perform the first successful heart trans-plant in 1967 (see pages 190–93). Modern heart-lung machines use a high-performance microporous hollow-fiber oxygenator that allows for much more efficient uptake of oxygen into the blood.

Cryonics

Believers in cryonics think that bodies frozen in liquid nitrogen immediately after death will be capable of revival in the future using technologies not yet known to modern science. Several books proposed it in the early 1960s and in 1967 Dr. James Bedford became the first human to be cryonically frozen. Skeptics argue that it will be impossible to repair the tissue damage caused by long-term freezing and oxygen starvation, and that there is no proof that a revived person would retain their memories, cognitive function and personality. Human embryos frozen in fertility clinics, then defrosted and implanted in the uterus, have grown up to be normal human beings, but freezing someone who has already died is another matter entirely.

Willem Kolff's Artificial Kidney

LOCATION: Kampen, Netherlands
DATE: 1943
FIELD: Hematology, nephrology, bioengineering

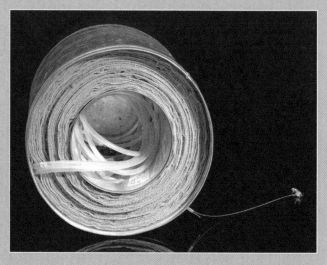

A range of diseases and injuries can cause the kidneys to fail, leading to a buildup of toxic substances in the blood, which disrupts the pH balance and causes edema. Before World War II kidney failure was almost always fatal but one man, Dr. Willem Kolff, working in Nazi-occupied Holland, managed to create the world's first artificial kidney. He did not have many resources at his disposal but built his first machine from old car and washing-machine parts, orange-juice cans and sausage skins. In 1945 it saved the life of a woman who was in a coma due to kidney failure, and heralded a new era in medicine in which machines could do at least some of the work of organs.

> *Dr. Kolff was a visionary who could see farther down the road than most of us ... One thing he did always amazed me: He could come to meetings, see a new procedure or material, then bring it into the lab and find an application for it.*
>
> —DR. DON OLSEN, PRESIDENT OF THE UTAH ARTIFICIAL HEART INSTITUTE, QUOTED IN *INTERNATIONAL NEW YORK TIMES*, 2009

CLEANING THE BLOOD

The kidneys are filters that remove waste products such as urea and creatinine from the blood, along with excess water and salts. They have an important role in blood pressure maintenance and also release erythropoietin, a hormone that stimulates the creation of red blood cells. About half of all cases of kidney failure are caused by diabetes, and about one quarter by hypertension. Other causes include diseases, such as malaria and yellow fever, or traumatic injury.

In 1914, a team working at Johns Hopkins University in Baltimore, Maryland, invented a "membrane vividiffusion apparatus" for dogs that separated particles in the blood according to their ability to pass through a membrane. The anticoagulant hirudin, produced by leeches, was used to prevent coagulation. There were too many problems to make human trials feasible at that time, so the research was put on the back burner.

In 1938 Dr. Willem Kolff watched a young man die a slow and painful death from temporary kidney failure and realized that if he had been able to keep the man's blood cleansed of waste products while the kidney healed, he would have survived. He began looking for solutions but his research was interrupted when German troops invaded the Netherlands in 1940.

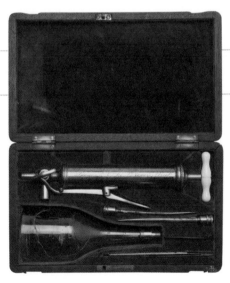

A History of Blood Transfusion

Back in the 1660s, the first human blood transfusions had such a high fatality rate that the practice was widely prohibited. In 1828 James Blundell used a transfusion to save the life of a woman with postpartum hemorrhage, and the procedure became easier in 1853 after Alexander Wood invented the hypodermic needle. It was still frequently fatal, however, and no one understood why until 1901, when Karl Landsteiner identified blood types A, B and O and realized that patients needed to be given the right type. In 1918 the first blood bank was set up in which blood could be stored for up to 21 days to treat soldiers in hemorrhagic shock after battlefield injuries.

James Blundell's 19th-century blood transfusion apparatus. He carried out 10 transfusions between 1825 and 1830, but only half were successful.

THE DIALYSIS MACHINE

Dr. Kolff moved to a small hospital in Kampen, where he could continue his research without collaborating with Nazi sympathizers. He used sausage skins as a membrane, filled them with blood, expelled the air, added urea, and agitated them in a salt bath. The small urea molecules passed through the sausage membrane whereas blood molecules did not, and within 5 minutes all the urea had moved into the salt water. Following this principle he went on to produce his first artificial kidney machine, in which 50 yards (46 m) of sausage skins were wrapped around a wooden drum sitting within a salt solution. The patient's blood was fed in and the drum rotated to remove the toxic waste products. To pump the blood back into the patient again he used the design of a water-pump coupling in Ford automobiles.

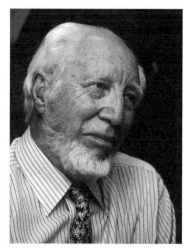

Willem Kolff, an extraordinary man who saved many Resistance operatives during World War II by helping them to simulate illnesses that required their hospitalization.

The first 15 patients on whom Dr. Kolff used his kidney machine did not survive but he made a number of modifications, including changes to the anticoagulants he was using, and in 1945 he saved a 65-year-old woman in a uremic coma. Many scientists would have patented such an innovation, but Kolff wanted to share his discovery and donated copies of his artificial kidney machine to hospitals in England, the Netherlands, Poland and the United States. Some doctors resisted using it at first, feeling it was unnatural to take blood out of the body, clean it and return it (a process known as dialysis), but soon it caught on.

At first it was simply intended to keep patients with acute kidney failure alive while their kidneys recovered, but during the early 1960s, Belding Scribner of Seattle, Washington, began to treat patients with chronic kidney failure by giving them repeated dialysis sessions. It was an expensive treatment in those days and patients had to come to the hospital twice a week for 16 hours at a time, but soon it proved successful. The first machines that allowed kidney patients to undergo dialysis at home were trialed in 1964.

One of Kolff's prototype rotating drum kidney machines. The first patient he successfully treated with it in 1945 was a Nazi collaborator, but he felt it was his Hippocratic duty to save her.

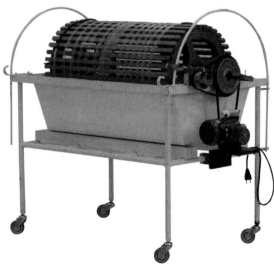

A large number of people react in negative way to anything that is new, anything they have not heard about before, that is not what they were taught, in school or in the university. I decided early that I would never be negative when I hear of something new until I have heard the full story, and have had the time to look at it.

—DR. WILLEM KOLFF, 1991 INTERVIEW WITH THE AMERICAN ACADEMY OF ACHIEVEMENT

KIDNEY TRANSPLANTS

Dialysis has drawbacks, because artificial kidneys cannot do all the work of real ones. They do not, for example, release erythropoietin, so dialysis patients often become anemic, and they are prone to infections. Kidney transplants are more desirable long-term and, because everyone has two kidneys, it is possible to use living donors. It is a relatively easy organ to transplant because it has just one main artery and vein. In 1954 Boston surgeons carried out the first human transplant in a 24-year-old man using a kidney donated by his twin brother, and the practice has become common since then, with a 5-year survival rate of about 90 percent.

However, kidney patients can face years of dialysis before a suitable donor kidney becomes available, and they may die in the meantime despite ever more sophisticated dialysis technology. Research is currently underway on an artificial kidney about the size of a coffee cup that can be implanted inside the body. This will contain a silicon nanofilter and blood pressure alone will force the blood through it. Stem-cell research (see pages 206–209) may also enable scientists to grow new kidneys one day.

Artificial Organs

Willem Kolff lived in the United States after World War II, and continued his research into all kinds of bioengineered machines that could take over body functions. He designed a new kind of permeable membrane for the heart-lung machine (see pages 168–71), and worked on the first artificial heart, which was implanted into a dentist, Dr. Barney Clark, in 1982. It contained a multilayer diaphragm designed by Kolff's assistant Robert Jarvik, so Kolff insisted, with typical modesty, that it should be named the Jarvik heart. Barney Clark lived only 118 days after the operation, but the experience took research a valuable step forward. In 1999 Dr. Kolff was part of the team that produced an artificial eye, and he also worked on artificial legs, arms and ears; his example inspired bioengineers all over the world to create machines to take over from other organs.

Trials are soon to begin on artificial kidneys that are implanted inside the body. These will filter out waste products and keep patients off dialysis without the risk of rejection that occurs with human transplants.

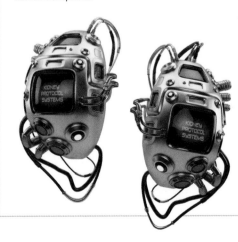

World Health Organization Flag

LOCATION: Geneva, Switzerland
DATE: 1948
FIELD: Epidemiology, public health

From the mid-19th century there were a number of organizations monitoring the spread of infectious diseases, such as cholera, plague and yellow fever, and agreeing on quarantine and other measures to resist them, but they tended to focus on specific geographical areas. After World War II, Chinese and Brazilian delegates to the United Nations lobbied for a global body that would devise and implement truly international health initiatives, and in 1948 the World Health Organization was formed. Its stated goal was "the attainment by all peoples of the highest possible levels of health" and its flag was the UN symbol overlaid by the serpent-twined rod of Asclepius, the Greek god of medicine.

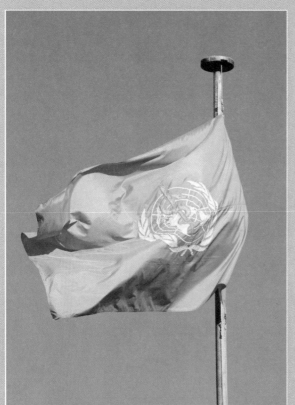

> Health is a state of complete physical, mental and social well-being, and not merely the absence of disease or infirmity.
> —WORLD HEALTH ORGANIZATION, 1948

SUCCESSES AND FAILURES OF THE WHO

The WHO's initial list of goals, drafted in 1948, set its top priorities as combating malaria, tuberculosis and venereal diseases; improving maternal and child health; and advising on nutrition and environmental sanitation. It launched an epidemiological service to inform governments of disease outbreaks, initially by telex and now via the Internet, and set up teams to advise on clean water and sanitation; the coordination and communication of medical research; and health advisory campaigns on subjects, such as nutrition, breastfeeding, smoking, drugs and safe sex.

Perhaps the WHO's best-known achievement was the eradication of smallpox in 1975 (see page 95), but its vaccination programs have also greatly reduced the global mortality from diphtheria, tetanus, whooping cough, polio, measles, and tuberculosis (TB), all of which were common causes of death beforehand. In 1955 it announced an initiative to eradicate malaria, but had to drop it in the 1970s, because it proved too ambitious. Its global polio eradication program had more success, with the number of cases reduced by 99 percent since 1988.

Detecting and reporting new disease strains is another extremely important aspect of the WHO's work. It tracks the strains of influenza and dengue fever virus each year so that appropriate vaccines can be created. It monitors the incidence of HIV/AIDS to identify any new trends in infection rates, and it mounts surveillance campaigns to keep watch over avian flu (see page 155), hemorrhagic diseases (see pages 214–17), and the old enemies of cholera, plague and yellow fever.

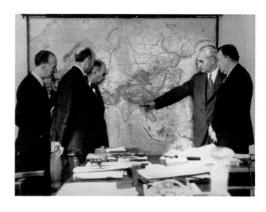

An interim meeting of the WHO in 1947, before its official founding date, to discuss plans for combating the spread of malaria.

According to Greek mythology, Asclepius, whose rod is shown in the WHO logo, was killed by Zeus for bringing the dead back to life.

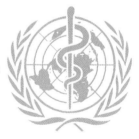

Living Longer, Healthier Lives

The work of the WHO has contributed significantly to an increase in global life expectancy since its initial formation. The average life expectancy of a child born in 1955 was 48; for those born in 2000 it was 66; and it is projected to rise to 73 for those born in 2025. The number of women dying during pregnancy and childbirth declined by 45 percent between 1990 and 2013, partly as a result of WHO campaigns, and the global mortality rate for children under the age of 5 dropped from 90 deaths per 1,000 live births in 1990 to 46 in 2013.

Crick and Watson's Double Helix

LOCATION: Cambridge, England
DATE: 1953
FIELD: Biochemistry, genetics

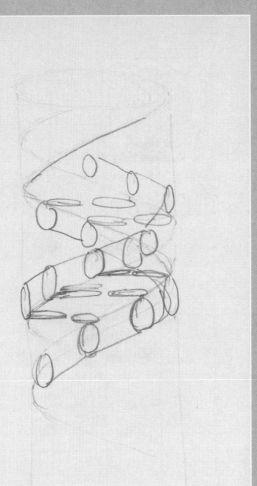

The double-helix structure of DNA—the substance found in every living cell that is responsible for passing on traits when cells reproduce—was not discovered by two scientists alone but by dozens of men and one woman working in different countries over the course of a century. The medical applications of their work are still unraveling, both in the fields of gene therapy and genetic screening. There are huge hurdles still to overcome, but it seems that in the future some congenital diseases may be prevented and many others cured as a result of the research of these pioneering scientists, of whom Crick and Watson are the best known today.

It seems probable to me that a whole family of such slightly varying phosphorus-containing substances will appear, as a group of nucleins, equivalent to proteins.

—FRIEDRICH MIESCHER, 1869

UNRAVELING A BIOCHEMICAL PUZZLE

DNA was first discovered in 1869 by Swiss chemist Friedrich Miescher. He was investigating white blood cells when he realized that the same substance existed in the nucleus of all living cells, and he called it nuclein. He was in no doubt about the significance of his find, but it was not picked up by other scientists until, in the early years of the 20th century, Russian-born biochemist Phoebus Levene began studying the function of nuclein. He found that there were two forms: DNA (deoxyribonucleic acid) and RNA (ribonucleic acid). He showed that DNA was made up of four bases—guanine (G), adenine (A), cytosine (C), and thymine (T)—a sugar called deoxyribose and a phosphate group; and that these were linked together in the order of phosphate–sugar–base to form units that he called nucleotides. An Austro-Hungarian biochemist, Erwin Chargaff, discovered two basic rules regarding this structure, known as the Chargaff ratios. He found that the amount of guanine (G) was always the same as that of cytosine (C), that the amount of adenine (A) equaled that of thymine (T), and that the relative quantity of each base varied from species to species.

Until the 1940s, it had been believed that complex proteins carried inherited traits from generation to generation, but Erwin Schrödinger suggested in his 1944 book *What is Life?* that such a function required an irregular crystal with no repetition in the pattern of its bonds, so it could hold an enormous amount of information. This was the key. It wasn't long before scientists realized there was enough complexity in DNA for it to contain coding, almost like Morse code, based on these G, A, C and T units.

Gregor Mendel

Gregor Mendel was an Austrian monk who established many of the basic rules of heredity while working in his monastery garden between 1856 and 1863 on hybrids of tens of thousands of pea plants. At the time it was thought that offspring inherited a blend of the parents' traits, but Mendel discovered that genes come in pairs and are inherited as distinct units instead of blended ones. He showed that there are dominant and recessive genes, and worked out that many traits were passed on randomly, according to the laws of statistics. His theories were scorned at the time, but by the early 20th century, scientists were recognizing him as the "father of genetics."

Mendel chose to experiment on pea plants because there were many different varieties, they grew quickly and they could be easily distinguished from one another.

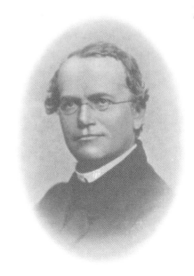

PHOTO 51

Between 1948 and 1950 at King's College in London, the New Zealand physicist Maurice Wilkins took x-ray diffraction pictures of DNA obtained from the sperm of a ram, and his studies led him to believe that the structure was a helical spiral. In 1951 chemist Rosalind Franklin was

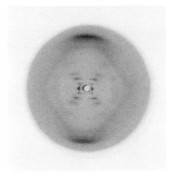

Photo 51: The dark patches at top and bottom show the four bases, whereas the arms of the cross show the planes of symmetry in a helix when viewed from the side.

brought in as a research associate to update the college's x-ray crystallographic laboratory, using techniques she had learned in her previous posting in Paris, France, where she had been studying the molecular structure of coal. The two got off on the wrong foot when Wilkins assumed Franklin was being hired as his assistant instead of an independent researcher, and their relationship continued to be hostile throughout the years she worked there.

Franklin began taking her own x-ray diffraction photos of DNA, refining and perfecting her work until in May 1952, working under her supervision, a PhD student named Raymond Gosling was able to get the clearest picture yet. The image, which came to be known as Photo 51, showed the double helical structure, with deoxyribose and phosphate molecules forming a "backbone" on the outside and the four paired bases (A, C, G, T) inside.

Rosalind Franklin came very close to determining the structure of DNA herself. Her early death meant she never realized how much the helical model created by Crick and Watson depended on her Photo 51.

Meanwhile, at Cambridge University, in England Francis Crick and James Watson were also working on the structure of DNA; but Franklin showed them that their 1952 model, with the backbone on the inside, must be wrong. In early 1953 American Linus Pauling

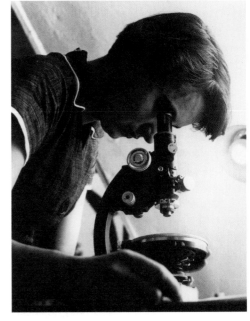

As a scientist Miss Franklin was distinguished by extreme clarity and perfection in everything she undertook. Her photographs are among the most beautiful x-ray photographs of any substance ever taken.
—J.D. BERNAL, OBITUARY OF ROSALIND FRANKLIN, *NATURE*, 1958

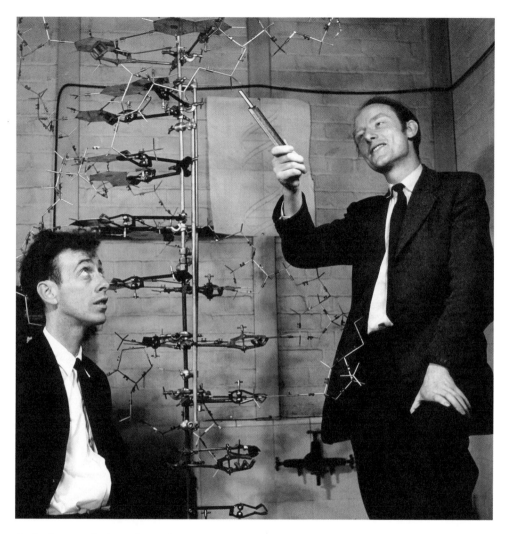

devised new techniques for making models, and Maurice Wilkins controversially showed Crick and Watson a copy of Photo 51 without Franklin's permission. She provided her numerical findings in confidence to a Cambridge colleague of theirs, and on March 7, 1953, Crick and Watson were able to produce their famous model of the DNA double helix.

The four agreed that Crick and Watson would take the credit for the model, although Wilkins and Franklin were credited with the background research. In 1962 the Nobel Prize for Medicine was jointly awarded to Wilkins, Crick and Watson; Franklin had died of cancer in 1958.

Watson and Crick with their famous model. They did not "discover" DNA, as is sometimes claimed, but used the research of other scientists to formulate the first accurate description of its double-helical structure.

The Double Helix

Each DNA molecule consists of two strands that wind around each other, linked by pairs of bases that look like steps on a twisting ladder. The backbones are made by alternating groups of sugar (deoxyribose) and phosphate groups, and they are connected by hydrogen bonds between the bases. Adenine is always paired with thymine and cytosine with guanine. The sequence of these bases determines the information required for building, growing and maintaining an organism. The outer edges of the helix have nitrogen-containing bases, which are exposed to allow hydrogen molecules to bond with them.

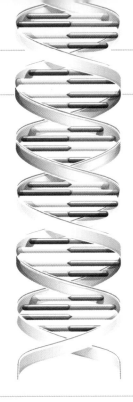

DNA molecules are wrapped around a type of protein to form chromosomes. Human beings have 23 pairs of chromosomes in each cell.

GENETIC ENGINEERING

Each human cell contains DNA that, when stretched out, would be more than 6 feet (1.8 m) long, and just ⅒₀ inch (1 mm) of DNA contains about five million paired bases. Genes are groups of paired bases, ranging in size from a few hundred to several million, which carry the information that determines traits. Mutations in these genetic codes can cause congenital diseases, such as hemophilia, or make us more susceptible to illnesses such as cancer or heart disease. Over the long term, mutations also occur as organisms adapt to their environment, a process known as evolutionary change.

After the structure of DNA was understood, scientists around the world began to look at ways in which the knowledge could be used, and one was by artificially modifying the genes of one substance to transfer desirable traits to it from another. Certain enzymes were found that could cut pieces of DNA from one organism and join them into another. In 1973 a cluster of bacteria became the world's first genetically modified organisms, followed by some laboratory mice in 1974.

One of the first practical applications of genetic engineering came in 1982, when bacteria were successfully modified to produce human insulin, which could be used by diabetics (see pages 156–59). Human growth hormones, antibodies, vaccines and many other medications have since been developed. Viruses can also be engineered to remove the infectious sequences and thus confer immunity on humans.

Genetically modified (GM) crops have been engineered to resist drought or pest attacks, and GM foods first went on sale in 1994. Laboratory mice have also been genetically engineered so they can be used for research into cancer, heart disease, aging and obesity. Pigs are being bred to grow organs that can be transplanted into humans, as well as for research into Parkinson's disease.

GENE THERAPY

Between 1990 and 2003 the Human Genome Project achieved the incredible task of mapping all the three billion bases that make up the DNA of human beings. As a result of this, scientists have been able to identify the genes responsible for some diseases, thus opening the way for treatments based on gene therapy.

In 1990 the first approved gene therapy trial in humans involved transferring a gene into the T cells of children with severe immuno-deficiency, but problems were soon apparent. There are difficulties with integrating new genetic material across the cell barrier, there is always a risk of rejection and several repeat treatments are required because cells undergo a continual process of division and reproduction. Specially adapted viruses, yeasts and bacteria have been developed as vectors to insert healthy genes into diseased cells, and nanotechnology could provide future delivery systems (see page 201).

Diseases that affect a single gene, such as sickle cell anemia and cystic fibrosis, should in theory be easier to treat with gene therapy. There have been promising results in a number of trials so far. In 2002 sickle cell anemia was treated in mice; in 2010 a patient in France was

Cloning

During the last 50 years, scientists have been able to make genetic clones of a number of animals by planting a mature cell from one organism into an egg cell that has had its nucleus removed. They allow it to develop in a test tube before implanting it in an adult female. In 1996 Dolly the sheep was cloned from an udder cell of a 6-year-old sheep, and in 1998 researchers in Japan produced cloned cows. Cats, dogs, deer, rabbits and rats have all been cloned, and a few scientists claim to have successfully cloned humans but to date there has been no independent corroboration.

The sheep named Dolly was the first mammal cloned from an adult cell as part of a project researching the production of medicines in the milk of farm animals. She died at the age of six, after producing six lambs.

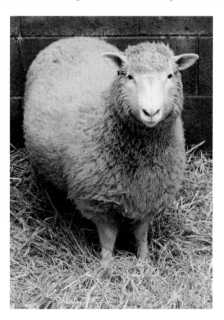

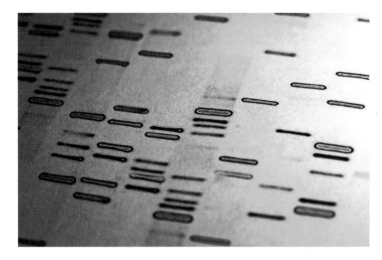

DNA profiling reveals each creature's unique DNA fingerprint. It can be used to establish familial connections, to identify criminals from minute traces left at crime scenes and to find gene mutations that could cause illness.

successfully treated for the common blood disorder beta thalassemia; in 2011 a pilot study of 59 patients with chronic lymphocytic leukemia saw 26 of them in complete remission after gene therapy; and there have been successful treatments of a number of eye conditions, including retinal dystrophy.

In 2003 China became the first country to license commercial production of gene therapy with Gendicine, a virus that treats cancers of the head and neck by entering the tumor cells and interfering with their genetic code. Russia followed in 2011 with Neovasculgen for treating peripheral artery disease, and in 2012 Glybera was licensed in the United States and Europe for treating lipoprotein lipase (LPL) deficiency, a condition that causes pancreatitis, by delivering an intact copy of the LPL gene.

In 2015 Elizabeth Parrish became the first person to undergo antiaging gene therapy in a program known as Strategies for Engineered Negligible Senescence, and the results are eagerly awaited. In the future, athletes could be given gene therapy to improve their performance and it could also be used to improve appearance, memory, intelligence, strength and all kinds of human characteristics.

> *The capacity to blunder slightly is the real marvel*
> *of DNA. Without this special attribute, we would still be*
> *anaerobic bacteria and there would be no music.*
> **—LEWIS THOMAS, *THE MEDUSA AND THE SNAIL*, 1974**

GENETIC SCREENING

The ability to screen for gene mutations raises many ethical questions to which individual countries, religions and other interest groups have been formulating their own answers.

- The technique of amniocentesis (sampling the fluid surrounding the fetus in the womb) has been in use since the 1950s to determine the health of the fetus and see whether mother and child have compatible blood types; but now genetic tests on cells taken from the uterus can identify medical conditions, such as Down syndrome, Huntington's disease and other chromosomal abnormalities early in pregnancy. This puts the onus on parents to decide whether they want to terminate the pregnancy.

- Newborn screening immediately after birth is now routinely offered. It can identify genetic disorders, such as phenylketonuria (PKU), which is treatable if caught early, as well as thalassemia, sickle cell anemia and cystic fibrosis, which are life-threatening if untreated.

- Tests can identify whether someone is the carrier of a genetic disease, which could affect their decision whether to have children and risk passing it on.

- Predictive screening can show if someone has a gene mutation that predisposes them to particular diseases. Actress Angelina Jolie found in 2013 that she had a mutation in the BRCA1 gene that gave her an estimated 87 percent chance of developing breast cancer and a 50 percent chance of ovarian cancer; so she took the decision to have a preventive mastectomy and oophorectomy.

There are many ethical concerns. If a patient undergoes genetic screening, would the results be kept confidential? Or could interested parties, such as employers or insurance companies, require screening and discriminate depending on the outcome? Such issues have taken medical ethics into uncharted territory in the 21st century.

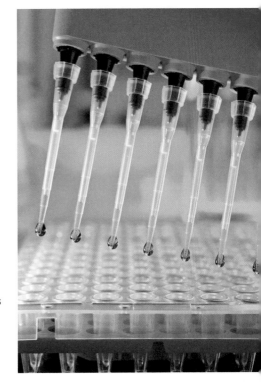

The polymerase chain reaction (PCR) is the most common technique used for amplification of DNA, producing millions of copies of a specific sequence that can be used in gene analysis.

Cigarette Package Health Warning

LOCATION: United States
DATE: 1965
FIELD: Preventive medicine

> *Smoking is a custom loathsome to the eye, hateful to the nose, harmful to the brain, dangerous to the lungs, and in the black, stinking fume thereof nearest resembling the horrible Stygian smoke of the pit that is bottomless.*
>
> —KING JAMES I OF ENGLAND AND VI OF SCOTLAND, *A COUNTERBLAST TO TOBACCO*, 1604

Hippocrates and Galen were quite clear that each human being had responsibility for his or her own health and that a moderate diet, exercise, sleep and fresh air were the best recipe for long life. Throughout the centuries when most diseases remained incurable, it was generally accepted that those who led a dissolute lifestyle could expect to die young, but with the medical advances of the early 20th century, this attitude began to change as we expected doctors to cure us. In the West, increasing numbers of people began to eat more food than they needed, drink more alcohol and smoke tobacco. When research showed that this was causing high levels of premature death, governments stepped in with preventive campaigns—among them cigarette package health warnings.

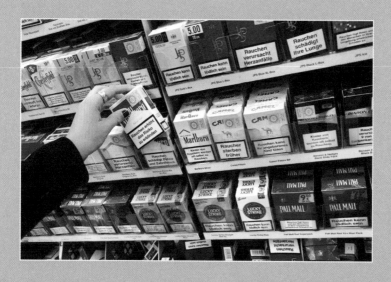

ALL THE SIGNS WERE THERE

There is evidence that tobacco leaves were chewed in the Americas as far back as the first century BCE, but the habit was only introduced to Europeans after 1492, when it was brought back by early explorers. The leaves were rolled up and smoked in pipes, as cigars or inhaled as powdered snuff. At first, tobacco was hailed as a general panacea for all kinds of ills, and in 1571 a Seville doctor listed 36 diseases that it could cure, including toothache, worms, halitosis—and cancer.

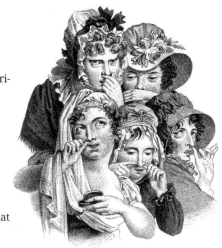

Women taking snuff in 1825. An article in The Gentlewoman *claimed that snuff could correct the eyesight, making eyeglasses unnecessary.*

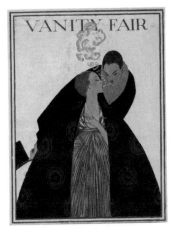

In 1604, King James I of England wrote the first antismoking pamphlet, *A Counterblast to Tobacco*. In it he warned that it unbalanced the four humors (see pages 26–29 and 37–38). In 1761 a London physician John Hill observed a vastly increased incidence of nasal cancers among users of snuff, and the antitobacco lobby began to grow. Disapproval of tobacco was especially strong in 19th-century North America, where it was linked with the religious temperance movement.

Left: During the early 20th century, women who smoked were portrayed as chic and daring, and role models included the fashion designer Coco Chanel and screen goddess Marlene Dietrich.

In 1912, American doctor Isaac Adler was the first to suggest a link between smoking and lung cancer, but still soldiers in both world wars were issued with free cigarettes along with their rations, creating millions of new addicts. Between the wars, tobacco manufacturers began to target women, promising them they would look more sophisticated and fashionable if they smoked, and some doctors recommended that female patients smoke to calm their nerves.

The Framingham Heart Study

This groundbreaking study began in 1948 with 5,209 healthy adults from the town of Framingham, Massachusetts; by following their health through subsequent decades, scientists were able to come to several important conclusions about coronary heart disease. Before the study it was believed that clogging of the coronary arteries was a normal symptom of aging, but Framingham scientists were able to show that obesity, smoking, high blood pressure and raised cholesterol levels (see page 191) increase the risk of heart disease, whereas regular exercise and a healthy Mediterranean-style diet decrease the risk.

THE EVIDENCE MOUNTS

Lung cancer was not recognized as a disease until the 18th century, and even in 1900 there were only 140 cases described in the medical literature; but the figures began to rise rapidly. By 1918 lung cancer was causing 15 deaths per million people in the United States, in 1930 it caused 49 per million and by 1968 it caused 900 deaths per million. All kinds of theories were put forward to explain this rise: asphalt on the roads, vehicle exhaust fumes, exposure to poison gas in the trenches during World War I, or the flu pandemic of 1918 (see pages 152–55), but gradually all the evidence began to point to smoking.

In 1939, Franz Müller of the University of Cologne in Germany published an influential paper entitled "Tobacco Misuse and Lung Carcinoma," in which he showed that people with lung cancer were far more likely to have smoked. Between the 1920s and 1940s, Ángel Roffo in Argentina demonstrated that it is tar instead of nicotine that is carcinogenic, especially the benzopyrene in cigarette smoke. And in a 1951 Washington University study, it was found that of 650 men with lung cancer, 95 percent had been smokers for 25 years or more.

The tobacco lobby was powerful, paying a lot of tax and employing a lot of people, but in 1962 Britain's Royal College of Physicians declared that smoking causes lung cancer; it was followed by the U.S. Surgeon General in 1964 and the World Health Organization (WHO) in 1970. In 1965 the U.S. Congress was the first national government to pass an act insisting that every cigarette package must have a warning label on its side. The first one read: "Cigarettes may be hazardous to your health."

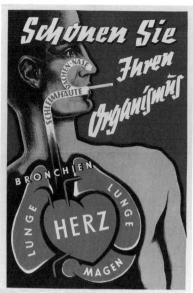

German poster, ca. 1900, showing the route inhaled smoke takes to the heart and lungs.

> *"Don't smoke" is advice hard for patients to swallow. May we suggest instead "Smoking Philip Morris?" Tests showed three out of every four cases of smokers' cough cleared on changing to Philip Morris. Why not observe the results for yourself?*
> —ADVERTISEMENT IN *U.S. MEDICAL JOURNAL*, 1943

THE EFFICACY OF PUBLIC HEALTH MESSAGES

The antismoking message was slow to get through, and many found it difficult to give up, but gradually the number of smokers began to fall in the West. In North America, 42.4 percent of those over the age of 18 smoked in 1965, but only 24.7 percent in 1997, with the rate for men (27.6 percent) higher than that for women (22.1 percent). However, as the market shrank in the West, cigarette manufacturers turned their attention to developing nations, where the number of smokers grew as dramatically as it had in the West in the early years of the 20th century. A 2009 survey in China reported that only 38 percent of Chinese smokers knew that their habit causes heart disease; and in 2010 in Vietnam, 88 percent did not know that passive smoking (inhaling other people's smoke) could cause heart disease.

Public health campaigns have been launched on a range of other issues:

- Road safety campaigns urged drivers to wear safety belts, not to drive under the influence of alcohol and to put children in booster seats; but statistics show that there was no fall in road accident deaths until after these measures became law and were vigorously enforced.

- Food safety improved enormously in the 20th century, with campaigns aimed at packing plants urging regular handwashing, safe refrigeration practices, pasteurization and pesticide use. Incidence of food-borne infections such as typhoid fever, TB, botulism and scarlet fever dropped dramatically.

- As late as the 1950s, it was not uncommon for children to die of measles or whooping cough, but immunization campaigns at national and global levels have reduced cases of infection and mortality. Between 2000 and 2014, measles vaccinations resulted in a global drop in deaths from measles of 79 percent.

- During the second half of the 20th century, fluoridation of water helped to reduce the incidence of dental caries.

Some may resent government intervention in matters of personal health, but all the evidence points to its being effective in the longer term.

Typhoid Mary

Typhoid fever is caused by consuming food infected with the *Salmonella typhi* bacteria from feces. Public health campaigns in the early 20th century encouraged handwashing after going to the bathroom, but Mary Mallon, an Irish-born cook in New York, didn't think she needed to bother, because she was not ill. After people began to become ill with typhoid at every house in which she worked, she was arrested and found to be an asymptomatic carrier (a person infected with a disease but showing no symptoms); she had a pool of typhus bacteria in her gallbladder. She was released from detention after promising not to work as a cook anymore, but she returned to work under another name. It is estimated that 51 people were infected by her cooking, three of whom died.

The much-publicized case of Mary Mallon helped to raise awareness of the need for handwashing before food preparation to prevent typhoid.

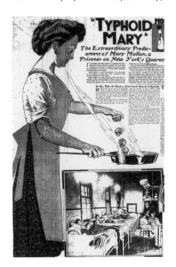

The First Heart Transplant

LOCATION: Cape Town, South Africa
DATE: 1967
FIELD: Cardiology, immunology

For a dying man it is not a difficult decision because he knows he is at the end .... If a lion chases you to the bank of a river filled with crocodiles, you will leap into the water convinced you have a chance to swim to the other side. But you would never accept such odds if there were no lion.

—CHRISTIAAN BARNARD, QUOTED IN DONALD MCRAE, *EVERY SECOND COUNTS*, 2007

Historically, the heart was seen as the seat of the soul, so the idea of transplanting a heart was shocking to many. All the same, 20th-century surgeons persisted in trying, because coronary heart disease had become the biggest killer in the Western world. A team at Stanford University seemed close to success in the 1960s, but they were beaten to the post by South African surgeon Christiaan Barnard, who performed the operation on a 55-year-old man in December 1967. The surgery was a success, the new heart worked, but 18 days later the patient succumbed to pneumonia. There were still many hurdles to overcome.

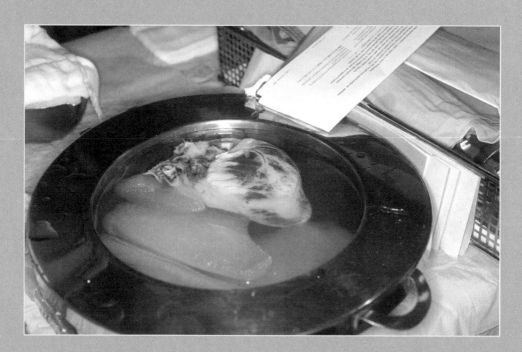

STEPS ALONG THE WAY

Several advances around the turn of the 20th century brought transplant surgery a step closer: German scientist Paul Ehrlich's discovery of antibodies, Austrian Karl Landsteiner's description of blood groups (see page 173) and Russian Élie Mechnikoff's research into the way the immune system works were all crucial in showing how a donor organ might be accepted by a new host. French surgeon Alexis Carrel developed new ways of suturing blood vessels in the early years of the century, and during the 1930s he collaborated with aviator Charles Lindbergh in developing a mechanical heart that could pump blood through the organs of animals, thus keeping them alive (see pages 168–71) while waiting to be implanted.

In 1933 American Frank Mann transplanted a heart into the neck of a dog and was able to keep it alive for 8 days. In 1946 Russian surgeon Vladimir Demikhov transplanted hearts into the chest cavities of dogs and they lived for up to 32 days. But still no one dared try it in a human.

Norman Shumway's team at Stanford University came up with a technique for cooling the donor heart to 50°F (10°C), and they designed a machine that could keep the recipient's circulation going until the new heart was ready to take over. Everyone thought Stanford would be the first team to perform a successful human heart transplant— but they were wrong.

THE FIRST HEART TRANSPLANT

One of the problems with human-to-human heart transplants was the need for a healthy donor heart that had not been damaged by whatever had killed its host. In January 1964, James Hardy at Mississippi Medical Center was planning to transplant the heart of a young man with irrecoverable brain damage into a 68-year-old man with advanced heart disease, but the donor was still not diagnosed as brain-dead when his

Atherosclerosis

In 1912 American James Herrick guessed that narrowing of the coronary arteries (atherosclerosis) was a leading cause of heart attacks. The first angiogram was carried out in 1931, using dye so that coronary arteries could be seen in x-ray and any blockages detected. In 1950 John Gofman discovered that men with atherosclerosis often had high levels of LDL (low-density lipoprotein) cholesterol and low levels of HDL (high-density lipoprotein) in their blood, leading physicians to advise patients that less animal fat should be consumed. Balloon angioplasty, invented by Andreas Grüntzig, was first used to repair a blocked artery in a human in 1974, and in the future nanobots (see page 201) may be able to do the same job.

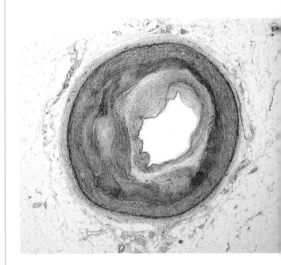

Artery showing atherosclerosis: Causes can include a diet high in animal fats, smoking, excessive alcohol consumption—and genes.

patient needed immediate surgery. Hardy tried implanting the heart of a chimpanzee instead, but it was too small to cope and the patient died.

Three years later, Christiaan Barnard, working at Groote Schuur Hospital in Cape Town, South Africa found the ideal heart donor: a 24-year-old woman, Denise Darvall, who had fatal head injuries from a car accident. Her relatives gave permission for him to transplant her heart into 55-year-old Louis Washkansky, whose own heart was failing. Barnard had studied Shumway's methods while doing postgraduate research in the United States, and he used them in a 9-hour operation on December 3, 1967. After the operation the new heart worked, but Barnard prescribed high doses of immunosuppressants to guard against rejection and 18 days later, with his immune system impaired, Washkansky succumbed to pneumonia. The operation was considered a success, because the heart maintained circulation until the end, but it

Xenotransplantation

In 1984 Stephanie Fae Beauclair was born prematurely with a severely underdeveloped left ventricle. Surgeon Leonard Bailey offered to perform a heart transplant using the heart of a baboon and her parents gave permission. The operation was initially successful, but baby Fae died 21 days later as a result of rejection. The case raised questions about the ethics of implanting animal organs into humans, a process known as xenotransplantation (from the Greek *xenos*, meaning "strange" or "foreign"). It had been around for a while. Back in 1838 the cornea of a pig was transplanted into a human, and between 1964 and 1977, sheep, baboon and chimpanzee hearts were transplanted into adults, all of whom died. Now it is thought that pigs are the most suitable animals from which to transplant organs into humans, and pigs' heart valves are often used to replace damaged human ones, although some object to this on religious grounds.

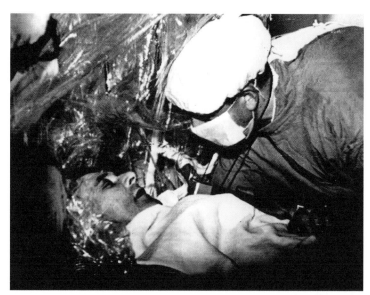

History in the making: Christaan Barnard with Louis Washkansky, who had experienced three heart attacks in the previous 8 years and was dying of heart failure.

was obvious that research was still needed on better ways of preventing rejection.

Other surgeons emulated Barnard's procedure and 100 heart transplants were performed in 1968, but none of the patients survived long. The number dropped to just 18 operations performed in 1970.

AVOIDING REJECTION

The breakthrough came in the 1970s when Belgian microbiologist Jean-François Borel created a medicine called cyclosporine from the fungus *Tolypocladium inflatum*.

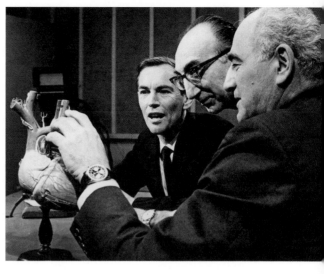

Christiaan Barnard (left) being interviewed on television in December 1967. He had been transplanting hearts in dogs since 1964 and in 90 percent of cases, the operation worked fairly well.

At first he was looking for a new antibiotic, but he realized that cyclosporine depressed the action of disease-fighting T cells without suppressing the rest of the immune system. It was the breakthrough that was needed to make transplant surgery work long-term.

In 1982, 39-year-old John McCafferty was given a heart transplant at Harefield Hospital in Middlesex, England, and at the time of writing (2015) he holds the Guinness World Record as the longest-surviving heart-transplant patient. In 1984 the world's first successful pediatric transplant was performed on a 4-year-old boy at Columbia University Medical Center. He needed a second transplant in 1989 but lived until 2006, when he died of other causes.

Since then, new combinations of antirejection medicines have been developed that can help to combat the increased level of atherosclerosis that often occurs with transplanted hearts. There have also been improvements in tissue-typing techniques to allow for better matches, but finding suitable donors remains a challenge. Approximately 85 to 90 percent of all heart transplant patients are now alive 1 year after surgery, with 75 percent alive after 3 years. Heart and lung transplants, first performed in 1981, are less common, but they now have an 85 percent survival rate after 1 year.

At that time, there was still a stigma attached to it. A big stigma. Actually, I think I was healthier after the operation than some people who have bypass surgery because I was completely cured. But when you mentioned "heart transplant," you got a very negative reaction. It triggered people's imaginations, and not in a good way.

—ROBERT ALTMAN, MOVIE DIRECTOR,
WHO HAD A HEART TRANSPLANT IN THE
MID-1990S, TALKING IN 2005

MRI Scanner

LOCATION: New York
DATE: 1971
FIELD: Physiology, medical imaging

It was eerie. I saw myself in that machine. I never thought my work would come to this.

—PROFESSOR ISIDOR RABI, WHO HAD AN MRI SCAN IN LATE 1987, ALMOST 30 YEARS AFTER HE DISCOVERED NUCLEAR MAGNETIC RESONANCE

During the 150s CE, Galen's only way of seeing inside the human body was by peering into the wounds incurred by gladiators. From the 16th century, dissection of the dead was legalized but there was still no way of seeing beneath the skin of the living in order to diagnose ailments. Physicians' understanding of anatomy and physiology increased greatly in the 1800s, but it was the 20th century before technology was developed that would allow clinicians to view the inner workings of the body. Principles were borrowed from many different fields to create new types of scanning machines, and the magnetic resonance imaging (MRI) scanner was in many ways the culmination—but the question of who invented it would prove to be controversial.

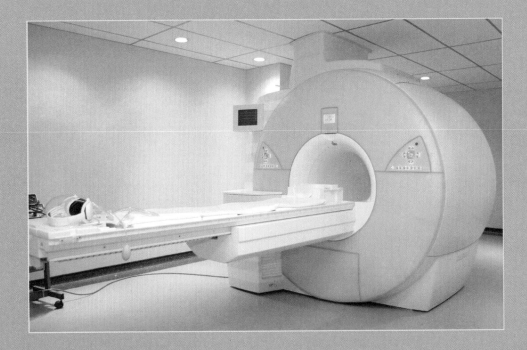

FROM X-RAYS TO SONAR

Röntgen's discovery of x-rays (see pages 132–37) meant that bones could be photographed and, when contrast agents were used, images could be obtained of blood vessels, the digestive system, gallbladder and bile ducts. However, the dangers of x-rays were known from the early years of the 20th century, and some patients were allergic to the contrast media, so other methods were sought for diagnosing diseases of the organs and soft tissues.

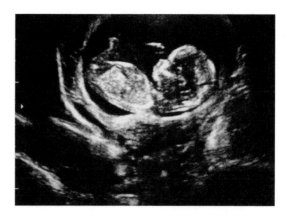

An ultrasound scan of a fetus at 13 weeks. Measurements taken at this stage can offer an assessment of the risk of certain chromosomal abnormalities, including Down syndrome, as well as help to date the pregnancy.

During the 1950s Professor Ian Donald of Glasgow University in Scotland created the first diagnostic ultrasound machine after watching sonar being used to detect underwater flaws in the metallurgy of ships. He initially used it to show abdominal tumors then applied ultrasound technology to pregnant women in 1957 to check for disorders in the developing fetus. Concerns that it could have harmful effects on babies proved unfounded and ultrasound is now used routinely during pregnancy.

In 1967, British engineer G.N. Hounsfield and South African physicist A.M. Cormack came up with a way of taking x-rays at various angles and using the cross-sectional views to build up a three-dimensional image. Computerized axial tomography (CAT) scanners originally took several hours to produce an image, but after they were speeded up, they became widely used to create detailed pictures of the inside of the body.

Positron emission transaxial tomography (PETT) was in use by the 1970s, when it was known as the "head-shrinker." Patients were injected with mildly radioactive glucose and, because different areas of the brain absorbed it at different rates, doctors could distinguish patterns that indicated illnesses such as schizophrenia, epilepsy and dementia.

Endoscopy

An early endoscope was discovered among the ruins at Pompeii, indicating that the Romans were curious to see what was going on inside their digestive tracts. In 1805 Philipp Bozzini of Frankfurt, Germany, used a tube he called the Lichtleiter (light-guiding instrument) to examine the urinary tract, rectum and pharynx, but all the early designs used a rigid tube, which must have been horribly uncomfortable for the patient. It was 1949 before Olympus of Japan developed the technology to add a miniature camera to the end of the tube, and in the 1950s fiber-optic cables were used to make endoscopes fully flexible while still able to take images of our insides.

WHO INVENTED MRI?

In 1882, Hungarian scientist Nicola Tesla discovered rotating magnetic fields, and he was honored by having the units used to measure the strength of magnetism named after him. Another 55 years later, Professor Isidor Rabi in New York showed that when placed in a magnetic field, certain nuclei absorb and then emit electromagnetic radiation. In 1946, Felix Bloch and Edward Purcell showed how this "nuclear magnetic resonance" could be used to measure the properties of chemical and physical substances, but it would be the early 1970s before it was applied to medicine.

A "Jedi" helmet used to take a magnet resonance imaging (MRI) scan of the brain, named after the Jedi knights in the Star Wars movies.

Raymond Damadian of Brooklyn, New York, discovered that when subjected to a strong magnetic field, cancerous tissue behaves differently from normal tissue. The magnetism causes hydrogen atoms to emit radio waves and, because tumors contain more water than healthy cells, they also contain more hydrogen, which makes the radio waves linger for longer. Damadian published a paper about his cancer-detecting machine in 1971 and took out a patent on it.

Meanwhile, Paul Lauterbur at New York's Stony Brook University introduced gradients into the magnetic field to determine the origin of radio waves being emitted, and was thus able to produce MRI images. The first pictures he took were of a clam his daughter had found on the beach, a green bell pepper, and two test tubes of "heavy water" (with extra hydrogen) in a beaker of normal water. The pictures were

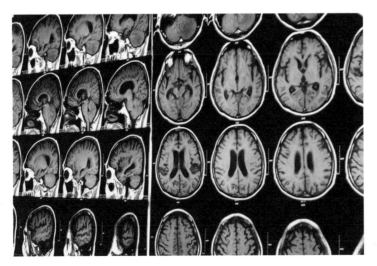

Computed tomography (CT) brain scans use multiple x-rays to build a 3D picture. They can detect tumors, stroke, bleeding and buildup of fluid in the brain.

fuzzy but the principle was one of the most important medical break-throughs of the century. English physicist Peter Mansfield developed a way of analyzing MRI images, and also devised echo-planar imaging to allow them to be produced quickly, making it a practical technology for use in hospitals.

In 2003, when Lauterbur and Mansfield shared the Nobel Prize for Physiology and Medicine, Damadian was furious. He took out front-page newspaper ads headed "The Shameful Wrong that Must be Righted," but the Nobel committee refused to change their minds.

APPLICATIONS OF MRI

Unlike x-rays, MRI scans are harmless and they can provide a 360-degree view from almost any angle. It is easier to tell the difference between diseased and healthy tissue in an MRI scan, but because of the expense of the machines, they are often used to confirm diagnoses made by x-ray or CT scans instead of being the first port of call.

MRI is used on the brain to detect strokes, swelling, tumors or the demyelination (damage to the protective sheath around nerve fibers) that occurs in diseases such as multiple sclerosis; they can also show which areas of the brain are active at any given time. When used to picture the heart, MRI can highlight defects, tears and the extent of damage caused by heart attacks; it can also give especially detailed pictures of the organs. The MRI scanner genuinely was one of the most important recent advances in medicine—no matter who was responsible.

> A team led by a neuroscientist, an anthropologist and a social psychologist found love-related neurophysiological systems inside a magnetic resonance imaging machine. They detected quantifiable love responses in the brains of 17 young men and women who each described themselves as being newly and madly in love.
>
> —EUREKALERT!, MAY 31, 2005

Dementia

As people live longer than ever in the 21st century, dementia is affecting increasing numbers, with 47.5 million estimated to have it in 2015. Current figures indicate that 19 percent of those aged between 75 and 84 are affected, and nearly half of all those over 85. There are several different types of dementia, and functional MRI scans, which show the blood flow in the brain, can distinguish them, although diagnosis can often only be confirmed in autopsy. Key signs of Alzheimer's disease are amyloid plaques and neurofibrillary tangles in the gray matter of the brain. Vascular dementia is caused by disease or damage to the blood vessels supplying the brain, and in dementia with Lewy bodies abnormal clumps of protein occur inside nerve cells.

Surgical Robots

LOCATION: Vancouver, Canada
DATE: 1983
FIELD: Surgery

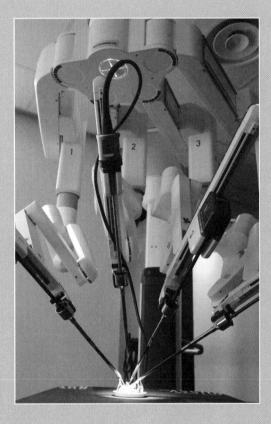

During the 20th century, there were huge advances in surgery as new kinds of scans enabled surgeons to plan operations in detail, and new instruments allowed them to work through smaller incisions using miniature cameras. The development of computers from the 1940s enabled the design of the first programmable robotic arm in 1954 and it was only a matter of time before this technology made its way into the operating room. "Arthrobot" was designed to increase the precision of hip joint surgery, and soon other robots followed, each with its own specialization and name, requiring surgeons to learn a whole new set of skills to work with them.

There's not a day that goes by that I don't think, "Oh my God; what am I doing?"
—DR. MANI MENON, HENRY FORD HOSPITAL, DETROIT, MICHIGAN, QUOTED ON NBC NEWS, 2012

KEYHOLE SURGERY

Open surgery on the abdominal or chest cavity requires an incision several inches long. This involves ligatures on any blood vessels that are cut, exposes tissues to the risk of infection and takes time to heal, leaving substantial scarring. In 1910, Swedish surgeon Hans Christian Jacobaeus performed the first laparoscopic (keyhole) operation on a patient's abdomen and the advantages were immediately obvious, but he was concerned about the risk of damaging tissues while being unable to see what he was doing. In 1919, Japanese professor Kenji Takagi used an approximately ¼ inch (7.3 mm) tube to examine the inside of a knee joint, and in the 1950s his compatriot Masaki Watanabe designed the first arthroscope, a small type of endoscope (see page 195) that could be inserted into a knee joint. The arthroscope allowed surgeons to see inside the joint and to remove damaged or torn cartilage through an incision of just a few millimeters.

In 1921 Carl-Olof Nylén of Stockholm, Sweden, built a surgical microscope for use in ear operations. Working through a microscope, surgeons were able to reconnect blood vessels and nerves of less than a millimeter in diameter, increasing precision and making many new kinds of reconstructive surgery possible. Microsurgery became much more common, because miniaturized tools were developed to assist surgeons and tiny cameras could project a magnified view onto screens.

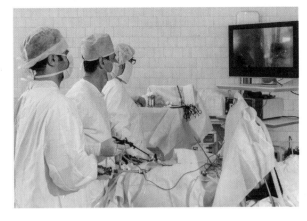

Surgeons performing keyhole surgery watch a magnified view on screen and move robotic arms to operate the surgical equipment.

ROBOTIC SURGERY

The first robotic arm was designed by Americans George Devol and Joseph Engelberger in 1954, and came into use doing repetitive tasks on a General Motors assembly line in 1962. Industrial robots were soon performing a wide range of tasks and it was inevitable that medical engineers would turn their attention to them in the ensuing decades.

Lasers

Einstein described the principle that led to Light Amplification by Stimulated Emission of Radiation (laser) back in 1917, but it was 1962 before it was first used in medicine, when dermatologist Leon Goldman employed a laser to remove a patient's tattoo. Many surgical uses have since been developed. Lasers can act as a scalpel to cut through tissue, they can vaporize soft tissues, such as tumors, that have a high water content, they can rejoin blood vessels and are also used in plastic surgery to remove molecular bonds in order to reduce wrinkles. Lasers are particularly common in eye surgery, for repairing detached retinas, removing cataracts and relieving glaucoma.

The original Arthrobot was designed in Vancouver by Dr. James McEwen and Geof Auchinleck, working in conjunction with orthopedic surgeon Brian Day, and it was first used in 1983 to solve a problem that surgeons confronted during hip replacements and arthroplasties (in which damaged tissue is removed from inside hip joints). The surfaces of the head of the femur and the acetabulum cup have to fit snugly together, but when adjusted manually there were often gaps that affected the patient's gait. Arthrobot was mounted on the femur, from where it ground out the joint surfaces along a preprogrammed path to achieve a perfect fit.

Other surgical robots followed. In 1985, PUMA 560 was used to position a needle in order to take a biopsy from the brain, guided by CT scans; in 1988, PROBOT was used to perform prostate surgery at Imperial College, London; in 1994 AESOP, a voice-activated robot, was programmed to maneuver an endoscope inside the patient during surgery; and in 1998 Da Vinci assisted during a heart bypass in Leipzig, Germany.

Instead of using one large incision to reach diseased tissues, robots typically rely on a number of ³⁄₁₆–³⁄₈ inch (5–10 mm) incisions around the site, into which small scopes or instruments can be inserted. They work with computer-programmed precision without any vibration from

> *We've found that younger surgeons who have experience with video games picked it up quicker than older surgeons.*
> —DR. MICHAEL PALESE, UROLOGICAL SURGEON AT MOUNT SINAI HOSPITAL, NEW YORK, 2012

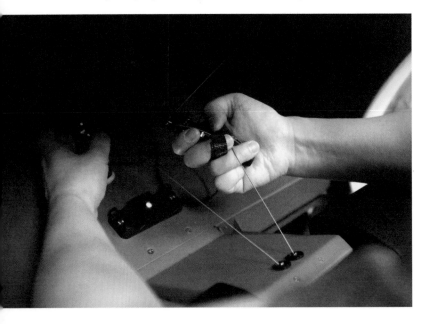

Hand controls with which a surgeon operates a Da Vinci robot. The machines can help surgeons to work in areas of the body that were previously difficult to reach. A Da Vinci robot typically has four arms, three of which can hold tools and is operated by a surgeon at a console. It is now used for prostate removal, cardiac valve and gynecological surgery.

machinery or from the shaking of a surgeon's hand, thus reducing the amount of tissue trauma. There is far less blood loss than with open surgery, less postoperative pain and recovery time tends to be faster.

Robotic surgery is now commonly used for unblocking arteries in peripheral artery disease, for gynecological surgery, prostate operations and to treat cancerous tumors in a range of locations by cutting off the blood supply and/or inserting beads of radiation, as well as in a range of heart operations.

REMOTE SURGERY

As robotic technology advanced, the surgeon did not even have to be in the operating room to perform an operation. In supervisory controlled robotic surgery, the procedure is carried out entirely by the robot following a computer program installed beforehand by the surgeon. In telesurgical surgery, the surgeon manipulates the robotic arms from a remote location (which can be either in the same room or elsewhere), using two foot pedals and two hand controllers, while watching proceedings on a three-dimensional screen. And in shared control, the surgeon carries out the operation while using the robot as a steady hand for miniaturized procedures.

In 2001, an operation was carried out across several thousand miles, with a team of surgeons in New York removing gallstones from a patient in Strasbourg, France, using a Zeus surgical robot and a high-speed fiber-optic system. This raises the possibility that in the developing world, where there are fewer hospitals and a lack of qualified surgeons, operations could be carried out remotely from one central hospital on patients in village health centers many hundreds of miles away. In wartime, surgeons could operate from a safe distance on soldiers injured at the front line. It also means that the most in-demand surgeons will be able to perform more operations, and they will be able to work anywhere in the world without leaving their hometown.

Nanotechnology

At a lecture in 1959, Richard Feynman predicted that one day we would "make machines at a nano-scale" that would "arrange the atoms the way we want." In the 21st century, nanotechnology has many potential applications in medicine, allowing physicians to make adjustments to the body at atomic or molecular levels. It's early days yet, but we can anticipate nanobots that perform surgery to disperse blood clots and repair damaged tissues at the cellular level; nanosensors that can diagnose diseases, such as cancer, at an early stage when just a few cells have mutated; nanosponges that absorb toxins; and delivery nanosystems that take smart drugs directly to the cells where they are needed.

AIDS Awareness Ribbon

LOCATION: Worldwide
DATE: 20th–21st centuries
FIELD: Epidemiology, virology

In June 1981, five men in San Francisco were diagnosed with *Pneumocystis jirovecii*, an extremely rare form of pneumonia. All were homosexual and all had severely compromised immune systems. The U.S. Centers for Disease Control and Prevention at first called the syndrome "gay-related immune disease" and the stigmatization of patients began, fueled by tabloid headlines about a "gay plague." It soon transpired that intravenous drug users were also being infected, as were those who had received contaminated blood transfusions, but the stigma remained. The battle to educate the public on effective measures to prevent the disease would have to scale a mountain of prejudice and misinformation that was unprecedented in the history of modern medicine.

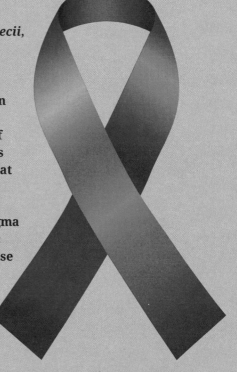

HIV does not make people dangerous to know so you can shake their hands and give them a hug. Heaven knows they need it.

—DIANA, PRINCESS OF WALES, 1987

THE ORIGINS OF HIV/AIDS

The virus responsible for the devastating disease appears to have originated in chimpanzees in West Africa, and been passed to bush hunters who came into contact with their blood in the early 20th century. The first human case researchers can reliably identify was a man in the Democratic Republic of Congo in 1959. The virus is not nearly as infectious as influenza, but it spread during the 20th century with the growth of cities across Africa, and a post-World War II vaccination program that used shared needles may also be implicated.

In 1969, the death of a St. Louis teenager puzzled doctors and tests on his remains in 1987 found he had been HIV positive, the first American confirmed to have the disease. After the 1981 San Francisco cluster, it was soon being diagnosed among drug users and hemophiliacs. In addition, Haitians, many of whom had worked in Africa, had a markedly high infection rate. It was clearly not just a disease affecting homosexuals, and it was renamed by the Centers for Disease Control and Prevention as acquired immune deficiency ayndrome (or AIDS). By 1994 it had become the leading cause of death among Americans between the ages of 25 and 44.

In 1983, a team at the Pasteur Institute in Paris, France, and a researcher in Maryland independently identified the retrovirus that was causing AIDS by destroying patients' white blood cells; it was given the name of human immunodeficiency virus (HIV). It was found that HIV could lie dormant within the body for up to 20 years before producing symptoms, and the enzyme-linked immunosorbent assay (ELISA) test to show whether it was present came into use in 1985. However, the challenge lay in getting people to take the test in societies where prejudice against those who were HIV positive was widespread.

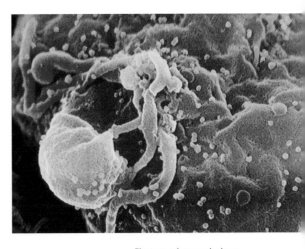

Electron micrograph showing new HIV cells (colored green) budding from a white blood cell after replication.

Misconceptions about HIV/AIDS

Among the early hysterical media coverage came suggestions that you could catch the HIV virus through kissing or sharing a glass with someone who was HIV positive. Some claimed you could get it from the seats in public restrooms, or from inhaling particles after a person with HIV/AIDS coughed or sneezed. In Africa, a dangerous myth was popularized that you could cure AIDS by having sexual intercourse with a virgin, and a number of churches worldwide claimed that AIDS could be prevented by prayer. Prominent celebrities who helped to dispel these myths included Princess Diana, who was photographed in 1987 shaking hands with an HIV-positive man. Actor Rock Hudson was the first major celebrity to admit to having the disease, 3 months before his death in October 1985.

THE HUNT FOR A CURE

By the middle of 1986, 21,000 cases of HIV/AIDS had been identified worldwide.

Without treatment, half of those who were HIV positive developed AIDS within about 10 years. After a diagnosis of full-blown AIDS, the prognosis was death within 6 to 19 months, as patients succumbed to a host of opportunistic diseases: Kaposi's sarcoma, a rare kind of skin cancer that caused raised blotches on the skin; cachexia, a rapid loss of body mass; pneumocystis pneumonia, caused by a fungus; and a range of bacterial and fungal infections that would normally be fought off by anyone with a healthy immune system.

The hunt was on to find a vaccine and a cure, but this proved difficult as the HIV virus was continually mutating. One researcher compared it to "trying to hit a moving target." AZT, available from 1987, was the first antiretroviral medicine used, but now a combination of two or three different drugs, known as highly active antiretroviral therapy (HAART), is common. This has made HIV a chronic but no longer fatal disease for those who can afford the expense of the medicines. It means that in the West, those with HIV have a more or less normal life expectancy; but in poorer countries, especially sub-Saharan Africa, where few can afford antiretrovirals, AIDS is still a major killer. Initiatives to find a vaccine continue; a drug called tenofovir disoproxil has shown promising results in preventing infection for those in high-risk groups.

The Death Toll

According to the World Health Organization (WHO), in 2014 there were 36.9 million people worldwide living with HIV/AIDS; 2.6 million of them under the age of 15, the majority infected by their mothers. As many as 19 million people may be unaware that they are infected, although in the United States, Russia and parts of Africa nondisclosure, exposure or transmission of the virus is now illegal. Most cases are in sub-Saharan Africa, but the infection rate is still growing in some parts of Latin America and Eastern Europe. Since the disease was first reported, 78 million have been infected worldwide and 34 million have died of AIDS-related causes.

Street art in Mozambique aimed at promoting use of condoms and showing the AIDS-awareness red ribbon. It reads: "Think of the consequences, change behavior, prevent HIV/AIDS." According to the WHO, 11.5 percent of the country's population aged 15 to 49 were HIV positive in 2015.

THE PUBLIC HEALTH MESSAGE

Early public health campaigns targeted homosexual men, urging them to use condoms, and intravenous drug users, who were encouraged to use free needle-exchange programs. Blood donors were routinely tested for HIV and blood products treated with heat to destroy the virus. However, public health officials were aware this was only the tip of the iceberg, because so many asymptomatic people could be hosting the HIV virus without knowing it.

In Africa it was seen that AIDS was killing equal numbers of men and women, and soon the incidence was rising among women in Europe and North America. It had to be made clear that the disease could be caught through vaginal, anal or oral sex. Mothers could pass HIV to their unborn children in the womb, during birth or during breastfeeding, so it was far from being the homosexual disease it was initially made out to be.

World AIDS Day is on December 1 each year and is a chance to campaign for public awareness and commemorate those who have died—more than 34 million of them since the virus was identified in 1984. The symbol of the red ribbon has inspired the use of ribbons for other health causes.

Sexual prejudice remained, however, propagated by fear and ignorance. In some workplaces, employees refused to work alongside those who were HIV positive, a situation dramatized in the Tom Hanks movie *Philadelphia* in 1993. Some insurance companies refused to cover people who were HIV positive, or even those who had taken an AIDS test, making people reluctant to come forward. In addition, the Catholic Church's stance against contraception was unhelpful, because condom use is one of the main preventive measures.

In 1991 a group of 12 New York artists got together to discuss a way of raising awareness of AIDS and signaling compassion for those affected by it. Their idea was simple but effective: a loop of red ribbon worn on the lapel. Within weeks, Hollywood celebrities were wearing them on the red carpet and the symbolism was universally recognized. At a 1992 concert in tribute to Freddie Mercury, the lead singer of Queen who had died of AIDS the previous year, 100,000 red ribbons were distributed and worn by the audience.

> *We live in a completely interdependent world, which simply means we cannot escape each other. How we respond to AIDS depends, in part, on whether we understand this interdependence. It is not someone else's problem. This is everybody's problem.*
> **—PRESIDENT BILL CLINTON**

Stem Cells

LOCATION: Madison, Wisconsin
DATE: 1998
FIELD: Biotechnology, cell biology, embryology

Back in the 19th century scientists realized that there were "ancestor" cells from which all other cells developed, and these became the subject of much curiosity and many experiments. It wasn't until the 1980s and 1990s, after new techniques became available for growing human cells in the lab and for altering genetic material, that it was possible to advance research on medical uses for these "stem cells." Today, they are thought to have the potential to repair tissues that have been damaged by hundreds of different conditions and cure many previously incurable diseases—but the research has not been free of controversy along the way.

> *Embryonic stem cells ... are, in effect, a human self-repair kit.*
> —ACTOR CHRISTOPHER REEVE ON *LARRY KING LIVE*, 2003

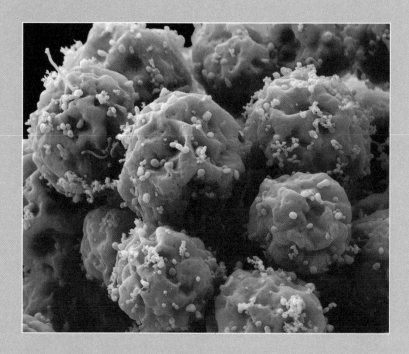

FROM ANCESTOR TO EMBRYO CELLS

German biologist Ernst Haeckel coined the term "stem cell" in 1868 to describe the original "ancestor" cell that reproduces to become an organism. In 1909 Russian Alexander Maximow discovered that all blood cells derive from one common stem cell in the bone marrow, which has the potential to differentiate into white cells, red cells, and all the other components of blood. Edward Donnall Thomas of the University of Washington realized that these stem cells could help leukemia patients, who have high numbers of abnormal white cells, and he attempted the first bone marrow transplant in 1957. His early patients died after their transplants were rejected but in 1968 the first successful bone marrow transplant took place, with a boy with an immune deficiency receiving healthy cells from his sister.

In 1981 Martin Evans of Cambridge, England, and Gail Martin of the University of California independently managed to isolate stem cells from mouse embryos, and they were able to develop an in vitro "stem cell line" in which these cells could be reproduced. And then, in 1998, James Thomson of the University of Wisconsin managed to derive the first batch of human embryonic stem cells from unwanted eggs obtained from fertility clinics. The potential uses of these were immediately apparent: for research, for curing all kinds of disease and to grow organs for transplant. However, in 2001 politics got in the way, when President George W. Bush vetoed a bill that would have funded stem cell research because it meant that a human embryo—albeit one that was never going to live—would be destroyed in the process.

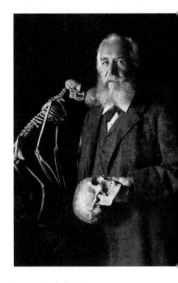

Ernst Haeckel was influenced by Charles Darwin's On the Origin of the Species, *published in 1859, and while pondering the concept of heredity became convinced that the nucleus of a cell contained information that affected its development.*

Cell Types

With the use of electron micrograph technology, researchers identified four different types of cells. *Totipotent* cells found in the earliest stages of development can go on to become any kind of cell; plant cells remain totipotent throughout their lives. In human embryos, about 5 days after fertilization a blastocyst is formed containing embryonic stem cells, which are *pluripotent*; they can go on to form all the cells needed in the body but not the placental or other external cells required for the organism to develop. Adult humans have *multipotent* stem cells in their bodies to repair and replace certain types of organs and tissues, such as skeletal muscle and blood. Unipotent cells, such as skin cells, can only reproduce themselves. Strictly speaking, only totipotent and pluripotent cells are true stem cells.

THE HEALING POWER OF STEM CELLS

With human embryo cells being scarce and their use controversial, researchers sought other ways of creating pluripotent stem cells. In 2006 Shinya Yamanaka of Kyoto University, Japan, managed to make embryonic-like cells from adult cells that had been reprogrammed by the insertion of four key genes. These were known as "induced pluripotent stem cells." Other researchers took the nucleus from a mature human cell and inserted it into an animal cell from which the nucleus had been removed, making a hybrid embryo that was 99.9 percent human. Others experimented with stem cells from the blood in the umbilical cord. In 2009 President Obama lifted the ban on funding embryonic stem cell research so that scientists could once again use human embryos, but there are tight rules surrounding such work.

> *Stem cell therapies have the potential to do for chronic diseases what antibiotics did for infectious diseases. It is going to take years of serious research to get there, but as a neurologist, I believe the prospect of a "penicillin" for Parkinson's is a potential breakthrough that we must pursue.*
> —JOSEPH MARTIN, DEAN OF THE FACULTY OF MEDICINE, HARVARD UNIVERSITY, 2004

If embryonic stem cells are allowed to clump together, they differentiate into different types of cells. The key was to find ways of directing this differentiation to produce the kinds of cells needed to repair or grow specific tissues. It seemed that many stem cells had a kind of homing mechanism that directed them automatically toward sites of damage, so they could potentially be used to treat degenerative disorders, such as motor neuron disease, osteoporosis, arthritis, Alzheimer's, Parkinson's and several kinds of eye disease. Where heart attacks or disease had damaged heart muscle, it might be possible to guide differentiation of stem cells into new heart-muscle cells. There are also many wheelchair users who hope that stem cells could help to grow new nerve cells that will help paralyzed people walk again. Unfortunately, such a development is too late for one supporter of this research, *Superman* star Christopher Reeve, who died in 2004.

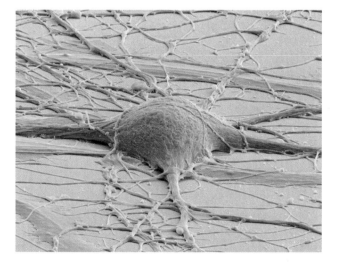

A neuron (human nerve cell) derived from an induced pluripotent stem cell, into which key genes have been inserted. These are currently used for testing medicines and could in future be used in transplants.

SUCCESSES SO FAR

Stem cell treatments are still in early stages. The most established use is in bone marrow transplants to treat diseases of the blood and immune system, but several other procedures have been trialed.

- Since the 1970s, skin stem cells have been used to grow skin grafts for burn patients, and it is thought that in the future hair and teeth might also be regrown.

- Stem cells have been used to repair damaged corneas but so far there has been less success in treating retinal diseases.

- Small-scale trials using stem cells to treat motor neuron disease have so far shown that they slow down the loss of neuron cells and may help protect existing ones.

- Researchers at Harvard University announced in 2014 that embryonic stem cells have been developed into insulin-producing beta cells in diabetic mice. Translated to humans, this would mean people with type 1 diabetes (see page 159) might no longer need to inject insulin.

Stem Cells and Cancer

Cancer rates have increased significantly over the last century, partly because humans are living longer. In 1997 a major study found that cancers occur because of problems in the differentiation process of certain stem cells. At present, cancer treatments destroy all cancer cells indiscriminately, but if it were possible to find the gene for the "cancer stem cells" in each type of cancer, medications could be developed to target them directly.

- Stem cells have been successfully used to treat tendon damage in racehorses and could in future be used for healing human tendon injuries.

- Autologous hematopoietic stem cell transplantation (AHSCT), currently used to treat leukemia and multiple myeloma, has shown marked success in treating patients with relapsing remitting multiple sclerosis. Of 123 patients tested, 64 percent reported being less disabled after treatment and 4 years later, 80 percent had had no further relapses.

- In 2015 fetal brain cells were used in the treatment of Parkinson's disease, but it could take years for results of this trial to become clear.

- Human trials to regenerate the spinal cord after injury are ongoing but there are no approved treatments to date.

Thought-Controlled Prosthesis

LOCATION: Gothenburg, Sweden
DATE: 2013
FIELD: Bioengineering, surgery, orthopedics

The oldest-known prosthetic device was a strap-on, leather-and-wood big toe found on an Egyptian mummy dated 950–710 BCE. Although probably designed for cosmetic purposes, it would have enabled the noblewoman to whom it belonged to walk more easily—unlike the clunky artificial legs made of iron that knights used in the Dark Ages. The technology of prosthetics advanced through the centuries, and in the 20th century new, lightweight materials improved both their appearance and their dexterity. In the early 21st century, researchers discovered ways to connect a prosthetic limb to the user's nerves, so that they could control movements simply by thinking. The first patient to receive an implanted thought-controlled limb was a Swedish truck driver (see below) in 2013, but many more have now been fitted, with highly encouraging results.

> *Reliable communication between the prosthesis and the body has been the missing link for the clinical implementation of neural control and sensory feedback, and this is now in place.*
> —MAX ORTIZ CATALAN, ONE OF THE PIONEERS OF OSSEOINTEGRATION, TEDX TALK, 2014

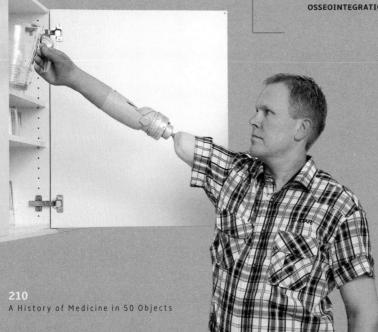

RESTORING FUNCTION

Losing limbs in battle was commonplace in the days of sword-fighting, and a few pioneering soldiers came up with their own solutions. Marcus Sergius, a Roman general who lost his right hand in the Second Punic War, used a hand made out of steel to hold his shield. German mercenary Götz von Berlichingen, who lost his right arm in 1504, designed his own iron prosthetic that could be manipulated with a series of springs and releases, making the hand open, close and grip objects. Pioneering French battlefield surgeon Ambroise Paré developed a number of improvements to prosthetics in the early 16th century, creating legs with knee-lock controls and fixed foot positions, as well as hinged hands. Many of his ideas are still used in prosthetics today.

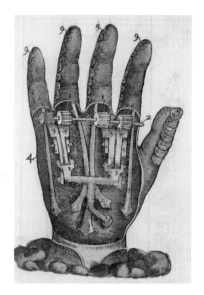

Materials for prostheses changed back to leather and wood, making them lighter, and systems of straps gave increasing control. The "Anglesey Leg" created by Londoner James Potts in 1800 had a wooden shank and socket, a steel knee joint and an articulated foot that was moved by catgut tendons, making it one of the most sophisticated of its era. Once anesthesia was used in surgery (see pages 98–101), surgeons could spend longer preparing the stump to connect with a prosthesis, and the bloody American Civil War, which created many new amputees, led to several refinements in prosthetic technology.

During the 20th century, advanced plastics and carbon-fiber composites made prosthetic limbs lighter, stronger and easier to control. External motors operated by switches or buttons could achieve tasks such as gripping objects, and computer-controlled knees could automatically adjust to the user's walking style. More advanced models could respond to the contractions of remaining muscles—but picking up signals from the user's nerves would prove more of a challenge.

Design for a mechanical hand by Ambroise Paré, 1564. During his 30 years as a battlefield surgeon for the French army, he devised many new surgical instruments and techniques (see page 125).

Left: The Anglesey leg was named after the Marquis of Anglesey, who commissioned James Potts to make it after he lost his own right leg at the Battle of Waterloo in 1815. At the time, most amputees used a wooden peg leg without articulated joints.

Athletes' Legs

The crescent-shape carbon-fiber legs used by Paralympic amputees, such as Canadian Earle Connor, have been accused of giving them an unfair advantage in races. Studies carried out between 2007 and 2009 claimed they can make amputees as much as 15 to 20 percent faster than they would be with normal legs. The blades weigh less than a lower leg, so athletes can swing them into position faster, and they leave their "feet" on the ground for longer, so they can push off with more force while using less muscular effort. The technology will probably improve every year, making Paralympic athletes run ever faster.

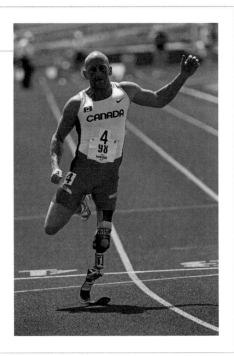

TOWARD THE BIONIC LIMB

During the 21st-century wars in Iraq and Afghanistan, improvised explosive devices caused a high rate of loss of limbs among service personnel and spurred researchers to design ever more sophisticated prosthetics. Dr. Todd Kuiken at the Rehabilitation Institute of Chicago developed a technique that he called "targeted muscle reinnervation," in which nerve endings at an amputee's stump are reattached to a healthy muscle elsewhere in the body; for example, nerves in an amputated arm might be attached to an area of chest muscle. When the patient thought about moving the arm, signals from the brain caused the chest muscle to contract. This was sensed by electrodes that provided control signals to the prosthetic limb, so by simply thinking of moving the arm, the patient could actually make it move. During a trial conducted in 2007 and 2008, all five of the patients on whom the technique was tried were able to perform a range of 10 different movements.

Brazilian scientist Dr. Miguel Nicolelis made significant progress on brain–machine interface technology. He and his team implanted electrodes in a monkey's brain that enabled it to control a prosthetic arm through its thoughts. In 2012 this technique was used on a 52-year-old quadriplegic woman, who was given a mind-controlled

Ninety percent of Paralympic athletes now use the J-shape "Flex-Foot Cheetah" prosthetics as worn by sprinter Earle Connor at the 2012 North/Central American/Caribbean & Canadian Masters Track & Field Championships.

prosthetic hand by a team at the University of Pittsburgh. Electrodes were implanted in her left motor cortex, the brain area that processes movement signals for the right side of the body, and after a few weeks of practice she was able to control the hand with her mind.

RESTORING FEELING

In January 2013, in a process the team at Chalmers University of Technology in Gothenburg, Sweden, called "osseointegration," seven neuromuscular interfaces were implanted into the upper arm of a truck driver who had undergone a below-elbow amputation more than a decade earlier. Before the operation he had been using a prosthesis controlled by external electrodes, but the connections proved unreliable and did not restore full function. After the operation the patient achieved enough dexterity with his prosthetic hand to enable him to operate heavy machinery at work and to tie his child's ice skate. He also experienced feeling in the hand as signals were sent back to the brain.

Soon after this, engineers at Johns Hopkins University in Maryland designed a "modular prosthetic limb," using 100 implanted sensors to pick up brain signals and control a robotic arm with 26 separate joints. The recipients were able to feel textures with their new hands, and in a test in which they were blindfolded, they could tell which fingers researchers were touching in 100 percent of cases. In a similar study in Rome, Italy, a blindfolded patient with a "bionic" hand could tell in 90 percent of cases whether he was being handed a ball of absorbent cotton, a plastic cup or a wooden block.

In May 2015 an Icelandic company announced it had fitted a prosthetic leg with implanted sensors. One of the great benefits of this is that it will force recipients to use their own muscles when walking, thus avoiding the atrophy that is a common problem for amputees.

At one point, instead of pressing one finger, the team decided to press two without telling him. He responded in jest asking whether somebody was trying to play a trick on him. That is when we knew that the feelings he was perceiving through the robotic hand were near-natural.

—JUSTIN SANCHEZ, U.S. DEFENSE ADVANCED RESEARCH PROJECTS AGENCY, 2015

Beyond the Wheelchair

In 2013 a robotic exoskeleton was launched that enabled users who had been paralyzed for years to stand and walk. Composed of a collection of batteries, sensors, motors, and microelectronics, it basically does the walking for the wearer. Technology moves fast in this field, and in 2015 a 26-year-old man became the first person with paraplegia from a spinal injury to walk without using manually controlled robotic limbs. He was fitted with an electrode cap that picked up brain waves when he intended to walk. These were transmitted to a computer that sent a command to a microcontroller on the patient's belt, which then stimulated nerves to trigger his own leg muscles to walk.

Protective Clothing for Ebola

LOCATION: West Africa
DATE: 2014
FIELD: Virology, epidemiology

> *It was clear to us that we were dealing with one of the deadliest infectious diseases the world had ever seen—and we had no idea that it was transmitted via bodily fluids! It could also have been mosquitoes.*
>
> —MICROBIOLOGIST PETER PIOT SPEAKING OF THE 1976 ZAIRE OUTBREAK OF EBOLA IN *DER SPIEGEL*, 2014

In December 2013, in a village called Meliandou in rural Guinea, a 1-year-old boy called Emile developed a fever. Three days later he died, the first victim of the most devastating outbreak of Ebola virus disease the world has ever known. Meliandou lies in a densely populated area near the borders with Liberia and Sierra Leone, and the virus spread rapidly. Medical teams came from around the world to help combat the disease, which had a mortality rate of about 50 percent, but despite taking precautions, health-care workers were succumbing. Their suits were cumbersome and uncomfortable in the stifling heat, and the slightest slip could prove fatal. A new design of protective clothing was essential.

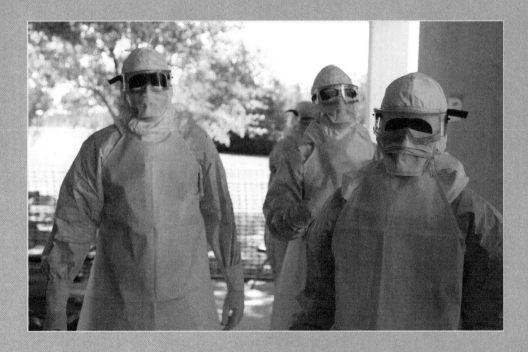

MARBURG DISEASE

In 1967, a team of researchers in the German town of Marburg imported some green monkeys from Africa to use in their research into vaccine production. Soon the team members became ill, with high fevers, diarrhea, vomiting and hemorrhaging from several different organs. Before the outbreak was contained, 31 of them caught the disease and seven died. The monkeys were identified as the source and a new, previously unknown type of virus was discovered, which they called a filovirus, because of its long, ropelike structure (*filum* is Latin for "thread").

Sporadic cases of Marburg disease cropped up over the following decades: in 1975 in Johannesburg, South Africa; in 1980 and 1987 in Kenya; then in 1998 there was a larger outbreak among miners in the Democratic Republic of Congo, in which 123 died. In Angola in 2004–2005, an outbreak killed 252, and showed a staggering 90 percent mortality rate. Many of the original victims had recently visited caves before becoming sick, and in 2009 the virus was found in fruit bats. This led to speculation that they act as hosts that are unaffected by the virus but can pass it onto other animals when they eat fruit on which the bats have nibbled. Humans then catch it from eating infected bushmeat (meat from nondomesticated animals).

In June 1976 a worker in a cotton factory in Nzara, South Sudan, became sick with hemorrhagic fever and died a week later; then in August a school principal died in Yambuku, Zaire (now the Democratic Republic of the Congo). At first it was thought Marburg virus was responsible for these outbreaks. A vial of blood from an infected nun was sent to a lab in Antwerp, Belgium, where a team including microbiologist Peter Piot discovered that it contained a filovirus, but not the one they had previously encountered. They flew to Zaire to observe on the ground, and chose the name for this new disease from that of the nearby Ebola River.

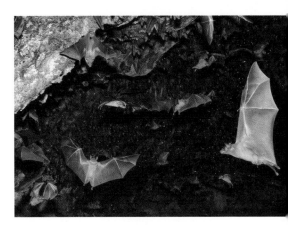

Egyptian fruit bats in a cave in Kenya: a common part of the diet in West Africa, bats could form a reservoir of ebola infection.

Diseases Named after Places

Zika virus is named after the Zika Forest in Uganda where the first case was found in a monkey in 1947. Lassa fever, a hemorrhagic fever transmitted by rodents, was first described in the town of Lassa in Nigeria in 1969. West Nile virus, borne by mosquitoes, was identified in the West Nile district of Uganda in 1937. German measles got the name because it was first described by German physicians in the 1700s. La Crosse, Wisconsin, and St. Louis, Missouri, both have types of encephalitis named after them, and Lyme disease is named for a town in Connecticut, where there was a widespread outbreak in the 1970s.

THE EBOLA VIRUS

Ebola is contracted by contact with the bodily fluids of an infected person. Flulike symptoms appear between 2 days and 3 weeks later, and these are followed by vomiting, diarrhea and hemorrhaging, as well as a rash in most cases. Initially, the virus is able to block the body's immune response, allowing viral strands to start replicating. These infect multiple organs, causing cells to die, and once the immune system detects those dying cells in the blood, it responds with a storm of cytokines (immune-system messengers that control the formation of blood cells and inflammation of tissues). The cytokine storm damages blood vessels, so they leak blood and plasma, and the cause of death is often hypovolemic shock from blood and fluid loss.

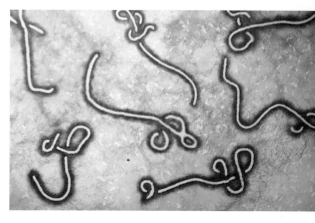

The Ebola virus has the threadlike structure common to filoviruses. There are five species—Tai Forest, Sudan, Zaire, Reston and Bundibugyo—and the 2014–15 outbreak was Zaire. At its height in October 2014, the virus was infecting 900 people a week.

Between 1976 and 2013 it is estimated there were 24 outbreaks of Ebola, affecting 1,716 people, but this could be a drastic underestimate because of the difficulties of diagnosing it. When patients present with high fever and diarrhea in central Africa, the first suspects are malaria and typhoid, and Ebola is only considered once there is a cluster of cases all experiencing hemorrhagic fever. Diagnosis is confirmed by lab testing, but this is not easy or convenient in the remote locations where the disease tends to spring up.

THE 2014–15 OUTBREAK

After Emile died in Meliandou in December 2013, he was closely followed by his sister, his pregnant mother and his grandmother. A traditional healing ceremony was held in which scores of household objects were burned, but the healer then succumbed to the virus. At her funeral, 12 women were infected after washing the body in a traditional burial ritual. It was March 2014 before Ebola was identified and reported to the World Health Organization (WHO), and by then there were cases in neighboring countries too.

Both Liberia and Sierra Leone were just recovering from civil wars in which their health-care systems had all but collapsed; Liberia had only 51 doctors in 2010, the rest having fled the violence. Existing hospitals

> *The hospital, especially the referral hospital, is the site where such outbreaks can either be recognized and halted, or unrecognized and disseminated. With them rests the responsibility for stopping the spread of these dangerous diseases.*
> **—WORLD HEALTH ORGANIZATION, 1978**

were totally unprepared for the barrier nursing required when treating Ebola patients. Health-care workers began to succumb, with an average of 10 percent of them dying during the ensuing epidemic. They had to wear masks, gowns, gloves and goggles to protect them from contamination with bodily fluids. Particular care had to be taken when removing the suits: one wrong move could expose them to viral particles on the outer surfaces.

New personal protective equipment (PPE) was designed specifically to help those nursing Ebola patients. The suits have built-in face masks and ventilators, and air vents in the hood help keep the wearer cool in hot climates. Crucially, a single rear zipper means the suit can be peeled off more easily, without the contaminated exterior touching the wearer's skin.

In February 2016 the outbreak has not yet been officially declared over because survivors can harbor small amounts of virus, causing flare-ups. It is estimated that 28,638 people were infected during the 2014–15 Ebola crisis and 11,316 died.

The Hunt for a Cure

During the 2014–15 Ebola epidemic, nine treatments were trialed, of which the best-known was ZMapp, but none have yet been licensed for general use. The most effective treatment was intravenous rehydration and careful monitoring of blood chemistry, but this was difficult to achieve in tiny local hospitals without laboratory facilities. In July 2015 researchers announced they had found a vaccine, VSV-EBOV, that seems to be effective and is now being offered to anyone who has been in contact with the disease. More conclusive testing will be needed before it is given to the general population in an attempt to prevent future outbreaks.

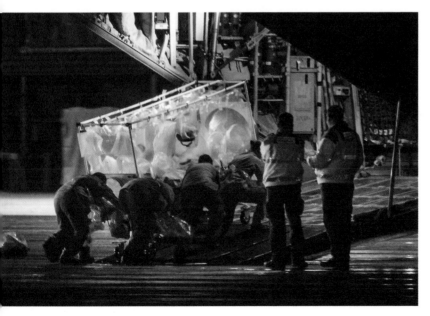

A quarantine tent cart containing a Scottish aid worker, Pauline Cafferkey, who contracted Ebola while nursing in Sierra Leone. She was declared free of the virus in January 2015, but 7 months later became ill again after a low level of virus in her brain triggered meningitis. She recovered, but continues to be carefully monitored.

Bibliography

Barnett, Richard, and Kneebone, Roger L., *Crucial Interventions: An Illustrated Treatise on the Principles and Practice of 19th-century Medicine*, Thames & Hudson, 2015

Bostridge, Mark, *Florence Nightingale*, Penguin, 2008

Brunton, Deborah, *Health, Disease and Society in Europe 1800–1930*, Manchester University Press, 2004

Bynum, William, *The History of Medicine: A Very Short Introduction*, Oxford University Press, 2008

Duin, Nancy, and Sutcliffe, Jenny, *A History of Medicine*, Morgan Samuel Editions, 1992

Elmer, Peter, and Grell, Ole Peter, *Health, Disease and Society in Europe 1500–1800*, Manchester University Press, 2003

Faherty, Anna, *Reading Room Companion ... acquired by and for Henry Wellcome*, Wellcome Trust, 2014

Kaptchuk, Ted, *Chinese Medicine: The Web that has no Weaver*, Rider, 2000

Lad, Vasant, *Ayurveda: The Science of Self-Healing*, Lotus Press, 1987

Mukherjee, Siddhartha, *The Emperor of All Maladies: A Biography of Cancer*, Fourth Estate, 2011

Persson, Sheryl, *Smallpox, Syphilis and Salvation: Medical Breakthroughs that Changed the World*, Exisle, 2010

Porter, Roy, *Blood and Guts: A Short History of Medicine*, Penguin, 2003

Revill, Jo, *Bird Flu*, Rodale, 2005

Shephard, Roy J., *An Illustrated History of Health and Fitness, from Pre-History to our Post-Modern World*, Springer, 2015

JOURNALS

Circulation, Journal of the American Heart Association
http://circ.ahajournals.org/

History Today
http://www.historytoday.com/archive

Journal of the International Society for the History of Islamic Medicine
http://ishim.net/newsletter.htm

Medical News Today
http://www.medicalnewstoday.com/

Medscape
http://www.medscape.com/

Nature
http://www.nature.com/index.html

New Scientist
https://www.newscientist.com/

Oxford Journal of Infectious Diseases
http://www.oxfordjournals.org/our_journals/jid/about.html

SOME USEFUL ORGANIZATIONS

Action on Smoking and Health
http://www.ash.org.uk/

Amputee Coalition of America
http://www.amputee-coalition.org/

Boston Children's Hospital
http://www.childrenshospital.org/
research-and-innovation

British Library collections
http://www.bl.uk/

Chemical Heritage Foundation
http://www.chemheritage.org/

Columbia University Dept. of Surgery
http://columbiasurgery.org//

Institute of Biomedical Science
https://www.ibms.org/

Microbiology Society
http://www.microbiologysociety.org/

National Center for Biotechnology
Information
https://www.ncbi.nlm.nih.gov/

Stanford Medicine News Center
http://med.stanford.edu/news/all-news/

U.S. Centers for Disease Control and Prevention
http://www.cdc.gov/

Wellcome Foundation
http://wellcomelibrary.org/

World Health Organization
http://www.who.int/en/

SOME INTERESTING WEBSITES

All About Robotic Surgery
http://www.allaboutroboticsurgery.com/
roboticsurgeryhistory.html

Antimicrobial Resistance Learning Site
http://amrls.cvm.msu.edu/

Big Picture
http://bigpictureeducation.com/

Braindecoder
https://www.braindecoder.com/

Brief History of Painkillers
http://io9.com/how-drugs-work-to-help-
you-ease-the-pain-1452216695

Chirurgeon's Apprentice
http://thechirurgeonsapprentice.com/

Explorable
https://explorable.com/medical-research-history

History Learning
http://www.historylearningsite.co.uk/

History of Malaria
http://www.malaria.com/overview/
malaria-history

History of Tuberculosis
http://www.faculty.virginia.edu/
blueridgesanatorium/tuberculosis.html

Internet Encyclopedia of Philosophy
http://www.iep.utm.edu/

Nursing and Midwifery in the Middle Ages
http://nursingandmidwiferyinhistory.
blogspot.co.uk/

Index

Page numbers in *italics* refer to illustrations

A History of Medicine in 50 Objects

Credits

Author acknowledgments: Grateful thanks to James Evans for commissioning me to write on such a fascinating subject, to Stephanie Evans for being the nicest, most efficient editor ever, and to the designer Lindsey Johns for making it all look so attractive.

Alamy/© David J. Green 25 (top); /© Mike Lester 26; /© picture 110

Photo courtesy of Alcor Life Extension Foundation 171

The Army Medical Services Museum, RAMC Muniment Collection. In the care of the Wellcome Library 150

Bridgeman Images 30

Creative Commons: CC BY-SA 3.0 31; CC BY-SA 2.0/Kim Traynor 51; CC BY-SA 3.0 136; CC BY-SA 2.5/Archives of Bayer AG 140; CC BY-2.0/Robert Huffstutter 142; CC BY-SA 2.0 146; CC-BY-SA 3.0 168; CC BY-SA 3.0 174; CC BY-SA 3.0 174; CC-BY-SA 3.0 181; CC BY-SA 3.0/ Nephron 191; CC BY-SA 2.0/Ton Rulkens 204; CC BY-SA 3.0 161; CC BY-SA 2.0 176, 177

Division of Medicine & Science, National Museum of American History, Smithsonian Institution 156, 158 (bottom), 159

Stephanie Evans 32

Getty Images: /BSIP 11; /DEA/A. DAGLI ORTI 41; 44; /Laister 161; /ullstein bild 170; /Universal Picture Archive 180; 183; /BSIP 190; 192; /Rolls Press/ Popperfoto 193; /François Guillot 198; /ChinaFotoPress 200; /Pacific Press 205; 217

King's College London 180

Library of Congress: 101, 105, 113, 123; /National Photo Company; 153; /Carol M. Highsmith 160; 187

Modern Art Foundation In Situ (Sokołowsko, Poland) 102

National Institute of Allergy and Infectious Diseases (NIAID) 167

Courtesy of the National Library of Medicine 6

Ortiz-Catalan et al., *Sci. Trans. Med.*, 2014 210

plantillustrations.org 59, 77, 86, 88, 90 (top), 99, 139

Public Health Image Library (PHIL)/CDC 61; /Cynthia Goldsmith 85; /CDC 154; /Shuqing Zhao, China 155; /CDC and C. Goldsmith 203; /Nahid Bhadelia, M.D. 214

Photo courtesy of Russian Academy for Medical Sciences/Lutfia Arifulova 169

St. Bartholomew's Hospital Archives & Museum/ Wellcome Images, London 129

Science & Society Picture Library/Getty Images 44, 108, 109, 138, 172, 173

Science Museum, London/Getty Images 5, 8, 14 (top), 72, 81, 82, 92, 98, 115, 120, 128, 134, 196, 211

Science Photo Library/Getty Images: /Steve Gschmeissner 206; /Thomas Deerinck, NCMIR 208

Shutterstock.com: /Monkey Business Images 7; /Mikhail Zahranichny 14 (bottom); /ileana_bt 17; /Vladimir Melnik 52; /Roberto Castillo 57 (top); /Marzolino 58 (bottom); /Alfonso de Tomas 66; / Everett Historical 78; /toeytoey 88; /thailoei92 134; 138; /Kalcutta 139; /steveallenphoto 124; /Everett Historical 152, 162; /Asianet-Pakistan 163; 165; /Everett Historical 166; /Ociacia 175;/Natsmith1 182; /isak55 184; /anyaivanova 185; /defotoberg 186; /Ezz Mika Elya 194; /fahrner 195; /Tushchakorn 196; /Beloborod 199; /olesya k 202; /Jamie Roach 212; /Ivan Kuzmin 215; /Nixx Photography 216

U.S. National Archives and Records Administration 127

Wellcome Library, London: 4, 6 (top), 9, 10, 13, 16, 18, 20, 21, 22, 23, 27, 29, 33, 34, 36, 38, 39, 40, 42, 47, 49 (top), 50, 54, 55, 56, 58 (top), 60, 62, 63 (top and bottom), 64, 65, 68, 69, 71, 73, 74, 75, 76, 77, 78, 80 (top and bottom), 81, 83 (top and bottom), 84 (top and bottom), 87, 89, 93, 94, 96, 97, 99 (top), 100, 104, 106, 107, 108, 109, 111, 112, 113, 117, 118, 119, 121, 130, 132, 133, 141, 144, 148, 149 (top and bottom), 151, 164, 177, 178, 179, 187 (right), 188, 196, 207, 211

Wikipedia/Jeff Dahl 12; 28, 154

All other images are in the public domain.